How to Stop Snoring

Liz Hodgkinson has been a newspaper and magazine journalist since 1967, specializing in the last few years in the health field. She has written many books, including *How to Banish Cellulite Forever*, *The Anti Cellulite Recipe Book*, *Smile Therapy* and *Happy to be Single*.

How to Stop Snoring

Effective ways to restore peaceful nights

Liz Hodgkinson

Thorsons
An Imprint of HarperCollins*Publishers*

For Ken

Thorsons
An Imprint of HarperCollins*Publishers*
77–85 Fulham Palace Road,
Hammersmith, London W6 8JB

Published by Thorsons 1992
10 9 8 7 6 5 4 3 2 1

A catalogue record for this book
is available from the British Library

ISBN 0 7225 2714 4

Typeset by Harper Phototypesetters Limited
Northampton, England
Printed in Great Britain by
HarperCollinsManufacturing Glasgow

Contents

Acknowledgements

The author would like to thank sleep and snoring expert Dr Christopher Hanning of the British Sleep Society, lung physician Dr John Stradling of Churchill Hospital, Oxford, Mr Michael Gleeson and Dr John Rees of Guy's Hospital, London, Dr John Woodcock of the Wythenshawe Hospital, Manchester, and Zachariah Evans of the Insomnia and Snoring Cure Group, for their help in preparing this book. Allen Davey, of the British Snoring and Sleep Apnoea Association, read through the manuscript and made many helpful suggestions.

Introduction

There are few prolonged tortures worse than being kept awake night after night by somebody who snores. You toss and turn, hoping against hope that by some magic the noise will die down and enable you to get back to sleep again.

If the snorer is lying next to you and is your husband, wife or partner, then at least you can wake him or her up and register your extreme annoyance. It's not so easy if the snorer is an elderly aunt in the next room, or a neighbour whose snores you can hear through the walls.

But even if you do wake up the snorer, it's not really a solution because you know that the next night and the next and the one after that are likely to be disturbed in similar fashion. Also, the chances are that as soon as the snorer nods off again, the terrible row will start up, as bad as before – while the snorer remains blissfully ignorant of it all.

In desperation, you may banish the snorer to a separate room, to the sofa downstairs, or leave yourself. You may resort to earplugs. You may even consider killing the snorer – the nightly nuisance can, at 3 a.m., lead to some truly homicidal thoughts.

Until fairly recently, snoring was considered a

menace only to those unlucky enough to be within earshot. Few people pitied the actual snorer.

But now, thanks to the intensive research which has taken place into sleep habits over the past 20 years or so, we now know that snoring is at least as bad for the snorer as for those who are forced to listen. The fact that he (and more commonly it is men who are affected) can't hear himself – usually – is beside the point, because chronic snoring is now known to be a medical problem, rather than just a nuisance.

Humans are not meant to snore, and when we do, this should be taken as our audible indication that something is wrong somewhere. The noise we call snoring is produced by vibrations in the throat and is caused by an obstruction of some kind, either in the nose or the throat. Of course, we all snore from time to time, such as when we've got a cold, after a heavy drinking bout or if, for some reason, we have fallen into such a deep stupor that we are breathing through the mouth rather than the nose and this is causing snoring.

Temporary snoring like this is nothing to worry about. It is when snoring is chronic and persistent, when it happens every night and when it gets louder and louder as the years go by, that it needs attention and treatment. Nobody should ignore snoring – and people who've been told that they snore should accept that they do, if only for the sake of their own health.

People tend to deny that they snore, even when presented with evidence in the morning from a tape recorder. 'How do I know it's me?' is a common defence. This is because, in the past, snoring has been seen as a trivial and embarrassing complaint – and also as something people could easily stop doing if they wanted to. Hearers have tended to assume that snorers do it on purpose, simply to annoy.

In the past doctors, too, have tended not to take the problem seriously. In any case, the majority of snorers would hesitate to mention their nightly habit to their doctor.

The trouble with snorers is that they always seem to be deeply asleep when they are snoring. But the fact is that all chronic snorers, however heavily they seem to be slumbering, will be suffering from disturbed sleep. Snoring actually constitutes disturbance, and not only to those within earshot. If nothing else, snoring tends to leave you feeling sleepy when you awaken. Anybody who snores and who lacks energy should assume that the two are connected.

Medical and scientific research has now shown that chronic snoring, if left untreated, can actually pose a serious threat to health. It can cause high blood-pressure, result in lack of oxygen to body cells and even, in severe cases, be a factor in strokes or heart failure. There is also a serious condition known as obstructive sleep apnoea, of which the main symptom is particularly heavy snoring.

One of the reasons that few doctors took snoring seriously in the past was that there were very few, if any, effective treatments available. Those days are over. Now, almost everyone who snores can find a suitable remedy or treatment which will ensure silent nights and blissful sleep.

The treatments on offer vary from simple lifestyle changes and cheap home remedies to high-tech breathing apparatus and surgical operations that have been specially developed to cure snoring.

It's all a matter of assessing your own snoring levels – or having them assessed for you – and then discovering the right remedy for you. Those who snore really heavily can have their sleep and snoring patterns accurately monitored in a sleep laboratory, and discuss the best remedy with an expert.

These days, sympathetic and effective help is available to snorers from the medical profession. There are also a number of patent cures on the market, and several of these have now been assessed in clinical trials and work surprisingly well.

Never imagine that you – or anybody within earshot – has to put up with snoring these days. It's all a matter of acknowledging and admitting it, and then making up your mind to get to the root of the problem.

To sum up, snoring is anti-social, a potent disturber of everybody's sleep, including that of the snorer, and a threat to health. It means that you are not breathing properly at night – and we now know that incorrect breathing sets up many bodily imbalances and health problems. Unless addressed, snoring will get worse as the years go by – and it will never go away by itself.

Snoring is *not* normal, it is *not* a joke, and it *does* constitute a risk to your health. So, whether you are a snorer, or unfortunate enough to live with one, don't just sigh and suffer. Make up your mind to take steps to stop the noise, for both of your sakes.

This book will help you to understand snoring – and tell you how to find the most effective treatment available.

CHAPTER ONE

Your Snoring Questions Answered

What Is Snoring?
The noxious noise we call snoring is produced by vibrations in the upper respiratory tract during sleep. It is caused by an obstruction to the airways of some kind, and is frequently connected with breathing through the mouth. This is why people tend to snore when they have a cold or blocked-up nose – they can't breathe properly through their noses.

When people breathe through the mouth, for whatever reason, air passages are dramatically narrowed. You can see how this works for yourself when awake if you lie down, then breathe with your mouth closed. The air should pass through without any trouble at all. Now hold your nose and breathe through your mouth. You will feel the soft tissues in the throat being pulled in as the air creates a vacuum. Breathing immediately becomes much harder work.

Although it is possible for humans to breathe through the mouth, we are actually designed to breathe through the nose. Mouth-breathing occurs when there is a blockage of some kind. The distinctive and highly unattractive noise known as snoring is produced by the collapsible parts of the throat – those parts such as the soft palate, uvula, tonsils and tissues around the

11

tonsils – vibrating because the passage of air is causing them to flutter. It's rather like a flag blowing in a breeze.

Noses are perfectly adapted to cope with breathing while we are asleep, whereas mouths are not. Anything that blocks the nose will put people at risk of snoring.

What Causes Snoring?

As a rule, anything that works to narrow the airways or causes partial blockage or obstruction when breathing can result in snoring.

It is now known that snoring can have a wide variety of causes. Some people will snore because of the anatomical design of their noses. People with long thin noses and very tight nostrils – the well-known British aristocratic nose producing the distinctive 'uppercrust' nasal twang – will tend to snore more than those with wide, flaring nostrils.

Snoring is very often caused by something being wrong with the nose. A deviated septum – where the piece of cartilage down the centre of the nose dividing the nostrils has become bent or twisted instead of straight, as it should be – can cause people to snore. People who have suffered some kind of injury to the nose, such as a riding or sporting accident, may subsequently snore.

Snoring can also be caused by nasal polyps, small nodules which grow on the inside of the nose. In fact, anything that causes a degree of nasal congestion can result in snoring.

People who have extra-large tonsils or adenoids have less space in the air passages and are therefore more likely to snore. Other anatomical reasons for snoring may be a long uvula and soft palate, which also have the effect of reducing the size of the airway and producing the fluttering effect in the collapsible tissues.

A receding chin can cause the tongue to protrude backwards and fall back even more than normal during sleep. Down's Syndrome children, for instance, are frequently snorers because they have large tongues which effectively block the airways during sleep.

Lying on your back while sleeping can cause snoring as the tongue is liable to flop backwards and the mouth drop open, causing partial blockage in the air passages.

Conditions such as hay fever, which cause nasal congestion, can result in snoring during the worst of the hay fever season. Any viral infection in the throat can cause snoring, but these conditions are usually self-limiting. Bacterial infections of the throat, however, or sinus trouble may cause persistent congestion and make breathing through the nose permanently difficult.

How Common Is Snoring?

We all snore now and again, but it is estimated that around 30 per cent of the adult population snores regularly. Around 50 per cent of middle-aged men snore, compared to around 13–14 per cent of middle-aged women.

Statistics assembled since 1968 in the USA – when the first statistical survey of snoring was undertaken – show that between the ages of 30 to 35, 20 per cent of males and 5 per cent of females snore regularly. By the age of 60, however, 60 per cent of men and 40 per cent of women are nightly snorers.

In 1983, an investigation undertaken in Toronto, Canada, found that 86 per cent of women said their husbands snored, and 52 per cent were bothered by this; 57 per cent of men said their wives snored, but only 15 per cent were troubled by it. This can mean one of two things: either that men sleep far more deeply than women – or that women's snores are less loud than men's.

How Loud Can Snoring Get?

Snoring levels of 80 to 90 decibels – the sound of a dog barking loudly – have been recorded. The world's champion snorer, Mel Switzer, whose excessively loud snoring has gained him a place in the *Guinness Book of Records*, has reached 87.4 decibels – the sound of a pneumatic drill, or a motorbike revving up right in your ear.

Extremely loud snoring can be heard from several rooms away, and in severe cases snorers find that they cannot easily stay in hotels, as guests in adjoining bedrooms complain.

How is Snoring Measured?

Diagnosing snoring levels is now becoming a more exact science, and there are generally agreed to be four basic levels:

Mild snoring is occasional snoring, usually when the sleeper is lying on his back or has drunk too much; *moderate* snoring occurs in all body positions and is frequent although not too loud; *severe* snoring can be heard from one or two rooms away; *heroic* snoring is extremely loud, can be heard from three or four rooms away, throughout the entire house, and possibly by the neighbours as well. The director of one sleep laboratory said that he had three referrals for one of his patients from neighbours complaining. 'Heroic' snorers frequently have to have double-glazing to keep the noise *in*.

Why Do Men Snore More than Women?

All surveys ever undertaken on snoring show the same result: male chronic snorers vastly outnumber female snorers. Most sleep researchers believe the main reason for this lies in the differences between male and female fat distribution. Men tend to have fatter necks than women, and snoring is closely associated with neck size. In fact, one of the first questions a persistent snorer will be asked is his collar size.

Fat around the neck is an outward sign of fat around the throat, and this can cause narrowing of the passages, making snoring far more likely.

Some researchers believe that male hormones, known as androgens, encourage excessive eating, weight gain and salt retention, all of which are associated with snoring.

It is also thought that the female hormone pro-gesterone protects against snoring to some extent by stimulating respiration. At any rate, women catch up fast after the menopause, although all the really champion snorers have been male.

Another reason – possibly – why men snore is because on the whole they drink more and because the

15

effect of alcohol on men is more exaggerated than it is on women. Heavy drinking is intimately associated with snoring. It is also associated with smoking, although as women smokers catch up and overtake men – there are now more young women than young men smokers – this difference might eventually disappear.

Around 23 per cent of the adult male population are not just snorers – but heavy snorers.

What Is the Connection Between Snoring and Smoking?

Smoke irritates the membranes in the throat so that they swell and restrict the air passages.

Why Does Snoring Get Worse as We Get Older?

The main reason for this is that the muscle tone of the tissues in the back of the throat slacken and get floppy with age. Also, there is a very strong connection between snoring and being overweight – and the typical snorer is an overweight, middle-aged person who takes little exercise and who always seems to be tired. As a general rule, fat people are more likely than thin people to be snorers and, as we know, weight has a habit of creeping up on us as we get older.

This is not, as was once thought, because metabolism slows as we get older, or because fat people have slower metabolisms than thin ones. In fact, recent studies at the Dunn Nutrition Centre in Cambridge, funded by the General Medical Council, have shown that fat people, on the whole, have *faster* metabolisms than thin ones. The plain fact is that weight piles on slowly over the years and we get into habits of eating too much. Excess weight is, as we know now, directly connected with overeating and has no other cause. Although some overweight people blame genetic inheritance, an under-active thyroid, or 'glands', the fact is that it's eating too much rich food all the time that causes weight to be put on – and snoring to develop.

Fat people snore more than thin ones because they have thick necks. Also, they tend to get tired more easily than thin people, because they have more bulk to carry round, and this means over-relaxation of the upper airway. Lack of exercise can be an indirect cause of snoring.

It's Said that Drink Makes You Snore. What Exactly Is the Connection Between Snoring and Alcohol Intake?

Alcohol depresses the central nervous system and leads to a deeper, more drugged type of sleep than would be normal and natural. The more drugged and relaxed the sleeper, the more likely the tissues in the throat are to become particularly slack, causing the noise we know of as snoring. It is the *effect* of the alcohol, rather than the alcohol itself, that causes the problem. One of the first lines of self-treatment in stopping snoring is not to drink any alcohol late in the evening.

Why Do We Snore Only When Asleep?

The main reason for this is relaxation. During sleep, all the tissues in the throat – plus the tongue and the mouth – are relaxed and not under our conscious control. During sleep, all relevant muscles slacken, the airways narrow anyway, and there is some resistance to breathing. This may or may not be enough to result in snoring.

Is Snoring Seasonal in Any Way?

Some surveys have suggested that snoring is far worse in the summer. The reason for this seems to be that more sun in the summer leads to more ultraviolet rays being absorbed by the body. This in turn leads to greater relaxation – and the more relaxed people are, the more likely they are to snore.

Can Any Drugs Contribute to Snoring?

It does seem that certain types of medication, such as tranquillizers, sleeping pills and some types of antihistamines, can aggravate snoring by deepening sleep and causing even more relaxation of the upper airway passages.

Is There a Connection with Diet?

Researchers are still divided on this one. Some alternative and complementary practitioners maintain that any foods that increase mucus secretion (such as dairy products) contribute to congestion and, therefore, increase the risk of snoring.

We do know, however, that overeating – whatever kind of food you take in – increases your risk of snoring by making you sleepy and fat.

Does Snoring Make You Less Intelligent?

As all chronic snorers suffer from disturbed sleep, it follows that during the day they are not going to be as bright and attentive as they might be. But people who snore really heavily night after night are also depriving their brains of oxygen, and this has been found to have a deleterious effect on their IQ, memory function and verbal fluency.

In an experiment conducted by the American physician Dr Jay Block in 1985, the heavier the snoring, the more the mental abilities of sufferers were affected. Almost all the people tested in Dr Block's survey were professors, people who needed particularly to be bright and alert.

Children who snore frequently *seem* dull. This is because persistent snoring means that they never really get a good night's sleep – and this of course affects their concentration during the day. As snorers are likely to be more tired than non-snorers, it follows that they will be less able to pay attention to what is being said.

It is also estimated that at least one in 11 road accidents are caused by people falling asleep at the wheel, and in many cases those involved in accidents will also be heavy snorers. In fact, a large-scale study carried out by British sleep expert Dr John Stradling, lung physician at the Osler Chest Unit, Churchill Hospital, Oxford, found that men who snore are six times more likely to crash their cars than those who sleep soundly.

The study discovered that three in every 1000 men aged 35 to 65 are at risk of potentially fatal car accidents directly related to their snoring. Therefore, falling asleep while driving can be a direct result of chronic snoring.

So, in addition to affecting intelligence adversely,

chronic snorers are a danger on the roads, both to themselves and other drivers.

How Is Snoring Harmful to Health?

The worse the snoring, the longer it has persisted, and the louder it is, the greater the risk to your health. We could say that *all* snoring harms health because anybody who snores regularly will have his or her sleep disturbed, whether or not he or she is aware of it. In fact, anybody who is persistently sleepy during the day and who also snores should directly connect the two.

Most ear, nose and throat (ENT) surgeons and experts on sleep now believe that snoring is not just a social annoyance but an actual medical problem. At the very least, it means that you are not breathing as nature intended, and this can result in going short of oxygen during the night – a cumulative problem which can lead to serious complaints in later life.

Snoring can cause high blood-pressure and heart failure. It is well known that persistent heavy snorers are more likely than non-snorers to have strokes. Continual blockage of the air passages leads to hyperventilation – shallow breathing – which, some doctors believe, is a prime cause of very many modern illnesses, including ME and allergies. The reason for this is that hyperventilation leads to too much carbon dioxide being blown out, which in turn affects every cell in the body to its detriment.

Most sleep researchers are now of the opinion that chronic snoring should not be ignored, but regarded as a potentially serious medical problem which needs attention sooner rather than later.

Usually, once a person starts to snore, the problem just gets worse and worse. It is unlikely that snoring will ever vanish of its own accord, unless of course it has been caused by a purely temporary blockage such as is caused by a cold or hay fever.

How Serious a Health Problem Can Snoring Be?

Snoring becomes very serious indeed when it is a sign of the condition known as *obstructive sleep apnoea*. Badly obstructed breathing can result in periods during the night when the sleeper actually stops breathing. The word 'apnoea' comes from the Greek meaning, literally, a cessation of breathing. Obstructive sleep apnoea (OSA) results when breathing is blocked to such an extent that no air flows through the nose or mouth despite efforts to breathe.

This cessation of breathing eventually wakes up the sleeper, who then struggles to breathe. His or her attempts are often accompanied by an 'heroic' snore. Oxygen levels then return to normal – but the sleeper does not feel refreshed from his sleep. Most sufferers from OSA wake up hundreds of times during the night, very often without realizing it – and then wonder why they are so very tired during the day.

There is another, related condition known as *central sleep apnoea*, in which the movement of the diaphragm has temporarily stopped. This type of apnoea, which is less common than OSA, is usually a sign of an abnormality in the part of the central nervous system that controls breathing.

Sleep apnoea is not just a health problem. Very many sufferers risk losing their jobs because they keep falling

21

asleep during the day and cannot seem to do their work properly. So snoring can also seriously damage your pocket and your job prospects, if it goes on for long enough.

Around 90 per cent of sufferers from sleep apnoea are men, and the usual profile of a sufferer is that he is middle-aged, drinks too much and annoys everybody by falling asleep constantly during the day. The problem is much more common in the US than in Britain, mainly because there are so many more overweight men who are also heavy drinkers there – although Britain and the rest of Europe are fast catching up.

As sleep apnoea creeps up gradually, like all health problems connected with chronic snoring, it has become known as the 'second wife syndrome.' When a man first marries, he is usually young and slim – and a non-snorer. As time goes on, he may start drinking and eating more and putting on weight. At the same time, he starts to snore. But as it happens over a number of years, his wife learns to cope with it.

Perhaps he then loses his wife or divorces. After a few years, he remarries. In the interim, his snoring has become steadily worse. His new wife tells him that she won't under any circumstances put up with the terrible snoring and that he must do something about it. So it is often only after the problem has been established for some years that treatment may be sought.

And although the sufferer may be reluctant to seek treatment – most snorers deny emphatically that they *do* snore (thus perpetuating the 'in the closet' aspect of the problem) – his second wife will be doing him an enormous favour. Because unless treatment is sought – and these days it can be extremely effective – a sufferer from sleep apnoea can become so short of oxygen during the night that eventually he dies of heart failure. In fact, single men who suffer from apnoea – and who have no one around to complain of their snoring – are far more likely to suffer from heart failure than men whose partners make them go for treatment.

How Successful Are Snoring Cures?

These days, very successful indeed. They range from the simple and cheap to the highly complicated and extremely expensive.

Anybody who snores – or who is told that he or she snores – should make concerted efforts to zap the nightly noise. Sometimes, simple lifestyle changes such as not drinking lots of alcohol or eating heavy meals just before going to bed will be enough to stop the problem. In other cases, though, snoring will need detailed investigation by an expert at a sleep laboratory.

Snoring can be related to a whole spectrum of problems, which is why it should always be taken seriously. Nobody should ever be ashamed or embarrassed these days to take a snoring problem to the doctor – the days when the only effective treatment available was earplugs for the long-suffering partner or family are over.

If simple measures, which will be described in detail in Chapter 4, do not work, then the next step may be referral to a sleep disorders centre. There are now a dozen of these in the UK, always attached to large general hospitals, and treatment is available on the

23

NHS. At a sleep disorders centre the doctor in charge – usually a lung physician – will take a detailed case history, try to assess the reasons for the snoring and recommend non-invasive treatment.

A persistent or heavy snorer, particularly where the problem has gone on for some years, may be admitted to the sleep laboratory to spend a night or two wired up to sophisticated machines. These will record every movement as the snorer sleeps, including his or her snoring levels. A lab technician will be in the next room all night, recording and interpreting data. All these instruments are non-invasive and the treatment is completely painless.

Most snorers spend one or two nights at the lab – one to acclimatize them and one throughout which they usually sleep peacefully. After all the data has been recorded, the doctor should be able to recommend the snoring treatment or cure most likely to solve the problem.

If the sleeper suffers from OSA, then the most likely remedy will be attending a Continuous Positive Airway Pressure (or CPAP, usually pronounced 'seepap') unit, which is very high-tech indeed, working like a vacuum cleaner in reverse by delivering air to the passages. Although CPAP units have been called the most effective contraceptive in the world – and you will see why if you look at the illustration on page 25), the improvement in quality of sleep and daytime energy is dramatic. Very often, the sleeper will feel wonderfully refreshed and raring to go after only one night on the unit.

CPAP units are not, though, curative, and will

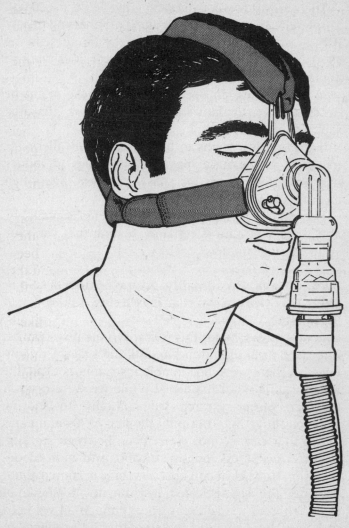

A CPAP unit

probably have to be used for the rest of the snorer's life.

There are also several operations available which will absolutely cure snoring. Uvulopalatopharyngoplasty (UPPP) is an operation invented by the Japanese in the 1970s expressly to cure snoring – and it does work in about 50 per cent of cases.

In some cases, an operation on the nose might be necessary, particularly where there is a deviated septum, or nasal polyps.

If the snoring seems to be caused by an allergy or irritation to the nasal passages, remedies to reduce the irritation, such as nasal sprays, are often recommended.

These days, a wide variety of treatments is available, and there will almost certainly be one that can cure your snoring problem.

People Have, Presumably, Always Snored – So Why Is it Only Now that it Is Being Taken Seriously?

One of the reasons for this is that serious investigation into sleep itself did not begin until the 1950s – mainly because there were no suitable instruments available for recording what happened while we were deep in slumber. Sleep research led naturally to snoring research, but it was not until the late 1970s and early 1980s that connections were made between snoring, daytime sleepiness, obesity, alcohol and high blood-pressure. Now, although not everything is known about snoring, the sophisticated instruments available in sleep laboratories can tell us pretty much all we need to know about treating and stopping the problem.

Is Snoring Getting More Common?

This question is almost impossible to answer, as scientific investigation into snoring is so recent. However, it would seem very likely that snoring is very much on the increase. Certainly, complications caused by snoring and sleep apnoea have become a huge problem in the US – and sleep laboratories have become a massive industry there.

Nowadays, we are eating more rich food, drinking more alcohol and taking less exercise than ever before. Although the benefits of diet and exercise have been extolled for a decade or more, it seems that relatively few people are taking any notice. Over 90 per cent of adults do no exercise of any kind after leaving school, and many find rich food hard to resist. It is certainly the case that more of us are regularly drinking alcohol than we ever did in the past. At the same time, the need to concentrate during the daytime, because more of us than ever before are in charge of instruments and machines that can be lethal or dangerous – computer systems, cars, aeroplanes – has never been greater. Dr William Dement, a pioneer sleep researcher in the US (founder of the first sleep laboratories in the 1950s and responsible for describing Rapid Eye Movement/REM, or dreaming, sleep) believes that many modern industrial accidents, such as those that occurred at Bhopal and Chernobyl, were caused mainly by daytime sleepiness.

So, whether snoring is actually becoming more common or not, the fact is that its consequences, both for individual health and for the safety of everyone, have never been more serious.

CHAPTER TWO

The Health Risks of Snoring

Until the 1970s, snoring was considered to be mainly a social nuisance, far more bother to the hearer than the snorer. There was very much a feeling that snoring was something that only exceptionally unloving and callous spouses inflicted on their partners. The implication was always: 'If you really loved me, you wouldn't snore so much.'

Also, if ever you wanted to convey that somebody was basically unattractive, or no good in bed, in spite of outward appearances, all you had to do was to suggest that he or she snored. There are few turn-offs more instant, and even the most wonderful romantic hero, the tallest, darkest, most handsome male ever to walk the planet rapidly loses his charisma if he is known to snore. Have you ever known a Barbara Cartland hero to snore? Can you imagine Daphne du Maurier's Max de Winter snoring? Can you imagine James Bond snoring, for all the champagne and shaken-not-stirred martinis he goes through in the course of an evening's seduction?

Of course not. Snoring is intimately associated with being undesirable and unattractive. And even though exceptionally loud snoring is known throughout the medical profession as 'heroic', few people would view a chronic snorer as being a hero, or romantic, or a wonderful lover. Snoring is one of the world's greatest anti-aphrodisiacs, and it turns sufferers into joke characters. Can you really take a man seriously if he is known to snore?

When I started researching this book, all kinds of women married to men I had considered successful, high-achieving and charismatic told me that their men snored – and instantly, the men in question were cut down to size. If I knew that a major political leader or media personality snored, it would be that much more difficult to take what he or she said seriously.

If a man is known to snore, his credibility plummets instantly. In literature, snorers are always played against romantic lovers: they are men you are not meant to take seriously, such as Sir Toby Belch in Shakespeare's *Twelfth Night* and the Fat Boy in Dickens' *Pickwick Papers*.

And if a snoring *man* is an instant turn-off, a snoring *woman* is even more so. Any beautiful woman who was known to be a snorer would instantly lose her charms. The Sleeping Beauty, for all that she was supposed to have slept for a hundred years, never became the Snoring Beauty, even though such a prolonged sleep would almost certainly have been punctuated (at least occasionally) by snoring.

So, given the bad press that snoring has always had, its close association with fatness, over-indulgence and undesirability, it's hardly surprising that people have been slow to admit to snoring and that the medical profession has been reluctant to take the problem seriously. For centuries, snoring has been regarded as a cartoon complaint, the butt of humour and satire, the curse of overeating and overdrinking.

It has been accepted for many centuries that snoring can drive hearers mad, which is the main reason so many patent cures have been invented over the years. Until very recently, all the anti-snoring treatments available were directed at stopping the noise, mainly so that hearers could get a decent night's sleep. There was little thought given to the possibility that snoring might be an actual medical problem, a signal that not everything was right with the system.

There was also little thought given to the possibility that snoring might in itself constitute a health risk, or that people with properly-functioning systems should not snore, at least on a chronic basis. Snoring was seen as a kind of curse on the unassailably unattractive, on those who could not control their appetites. Billy Bunter would have snored, along with being greedy, fat, sneaky, a liar and not very intelligent. But could you imagine Bob Cherry or Harry Wharton snoring? Never!

Snoring has always been, and continues to be, one of the favourite standby jokes of the cartoonist. A recent cartoon in *The Independent* newspaper, apropos of the film *In Bed with Madonna*, asked people queueing up to go into the cinema: 'Snoring or non-snoring?'

Even nowadays, because of the jokes and embarrassment surrounding snoring, people can be extremely reluctant to take their complaint to the doctor. All too often, even now, when most doctors will take snoring seriously, it is the wife or partner who complains first, asking, often in desperation: 'Isn't there *anything* you can do for his snoring – it's driving me mad?'

In the beginning, says Dr Bjorn Petruson, inventor of a nasal dilator to stop snoring, it is always the non-snoring partner who suffers first, having his or her nights broken and sleep disturbed by the noise. But as time goes on, unless the problem is taken seriously, it is the snorer who starts to suffer even more than the partner. Even if snorers do not develop a serious health problem because of the snoring, they will suffer from a dry throat, feel sleepy in the morning and become aware of their snoring as sleep is truncated and disturbed through increasing breathing difficulties.

The first and most difficult thing, often, is to get snorers to recognize and admit to the nightly noise. Most people vehemently deny that they snore – after all, they're not usually conscious enough to hear themselves, and as they would rather not snore they have difficulty believing that they do.

One of the odder facts about snoring is that although snorers succeed in waking up everybody within earshot, they themselves usually sleep apparently blissfully throughout the loudest noise. This is because snoring usually happens when people are very deeply asleep – and the deeper the sleep, the more likely the sleeper is to snore. The deep, drugged sleep that follows over-indulgence in alcohol is very often accompanied by snoring.

It is becoming increasingly difficult for snorers to maintain that they sleep quietly, however. It's easy enough for any member of the family to confront them with the evidence by leaving a tape recorder on at night.

31

In fact, one of the most important aspects of diagnosis for snoring is to have snoring levels assessed.

It's really only since the invention of the tape recorder that it has been possible to study snoring, as before, doctors had to rely on what partners or spouses said – and these might well have had a vested interest in exaggerating the noise.

Snoring, says Dr Christopher Hanning, an anaesthetist and president of the British Sleep Society, covers a complete spectrum of problems and always requires treatment – not just because somebody in earshot is complaining, but because snoring is always a health problem. We are not designed to snore or to have partial obstruction of the airways in the throat.

As snoring is not just a single problem, there is not just one treatment, and there never will be a simple 'anti-snoring pill'. Sometimes snoring may be caused by the anatomical design of the nose, sometimes by infection or nasal congestion, and sometimes it will have far more complicated and wide-ranging causes.

So far as we know, snoring is not hereditary. You do not 'pick up' snoring from your parents, or inherit a tendency to snore, although you may inherit the type of nose which predisposes you to snoring.

All snoring needs investigation. If you are thin, young, female and a chronic snorer, it is most likely that your snoring is caused by the anatomical design of your nose. This is not necessarily to say there is anything wrong with your nose, but that the way it is shaped means that air has a difficult passage through the nostrils. If this is the case, there are some simple devices, described in Chapter 3, which can solve the problem effectively.

If there's nothing wrong with the workings of your nose and you snore, there could be chronic nasal congestion. Again, this will need proper medical investigation.

Never ignore the snoring, or pretend that it's not happening. Snoring is not a character flaw – it is a physical obstruction and that's all. Very often, there will be a simple, non-invasive solution to the problem.

The main medical risk from snoring is that, at the very least, it makes the snorer tired. And increasingly, sleep experts believe that we are in danger of not getting enough sleep. Pioneering sleep specialist Dr William Dement believes that very many of our modern ailments and even psychiatric problems are intimately connected with a chronic lack of sleep.

Dr Dement is convinced that people suffer much injury, ill-health and depression because they just aren't getting enough sleep. Their current lifestyle, plus relatively modern innovations such as the electric light, videos and international travel, have led to a major reduction in time spent sleeping. He thinks that sleep deprivation is a prime cause of illness, poor performance at work and serious accidents.

Sleep-deprived doctors are, he says, a serious danger to their patients. Dr Dement is now trying to establish clear links between sleep disorders and physical disorders including hypertension, stroke and immune disorders. It is known that people with infections often 'sleep themselves better' and that those who can sleep recover far more quickly than those who can't.

It seems, from research, that we need around seven-and-a-half to eight hours of sound sleep in order to wake up refreshed and functioning. Few people can perform efficiently on less, and people who have less than four hours' sleep have a greatly increased mortality rate, according to figures released by the American Cancer Society.

British cardiologist Dr Peter Nixon believes that the majority of stress-related disorders, including heart disease, are caused by chronic exhaustion. Although not all British doctors share Dr Nixon's conviction of the close relationship between sleep deprivation and heart failure, sleep experts agree that sleep deprivation is the cause of more accidents and illness than most of us like to admit.

If you are snoring you are not getting a good night's sleep. Chronic snoring is an unmistakable sign that you are not breathing properly when asleep, and if you're not breathing properly for up to eight hours during the night, then it follows that your sleep will not have accomplished its proper restorative function. Any long-term disturbance of sleep will mean that you are operating at less than your best on a regular basis.

Improper breathing at night means shallow breathing, and this in turn can have the effect of the system going short of oxygen. This eventually affects the brain to its detriment, as well as every other cell in the body.

Above all, snoring is a cumulative problem, getting worse as the years go by, and causing ever more health problems.

Snoring and Hypertension, or High Blood-pressure

Snoring is associated with high blood-pressure because the blockages in the throat cause the amount of oxygen in the blood to fall when breathing in. This eventually places a strain on the heart and lungs, leading to high blood-pressure. Very often, people with hypertension are given tablets to bring their blood-pressure down.

But if they also snore, it may be better to get the snoring investigated first, to see if the blood-pressure levels fall of their own accord when the blockages are removed. It is better to have the snoring problem solved than to take blood-pressure tablets on a regular basis.

Snoring and Obesity

In popular literature and cartoons, snorers are always depicted as being fat. And although there are thin snorers, the fact is many people who are overweight may eventually become snorers.

But what is being overweight?

Nowadays, there is no guesswork about it. The way to calculate whether you are overweight is to look at the standard tables for height and weight as used by insurance companies. If you are 10 per cent or more above the standard weight for your height, then you are technically obese – and likely to encounter health problems because of this.

The fact is that we are not meant to be overweight – no animal in the wild is fat – and carrying around extra bulk does us no favours at all. Snoring is often the first sign that overweight is causing problems, as it means that too much fat is collecting round the neck (particularly in men, who are far more prone than women to putting on weight round the neck and chin) and causing a degree of obstruction in breathing at night.

If you are overweight, you are more likely to have breathing problems. When too much avoirdupois is accompanied by snoring, then it's time to take the two problems in hand. Overweight people find it more difficult to sleep on their sides – generally accepted to be the optimum position for sleeping, as it prevents the throat obstruction that can lead to snoring – and are also often short of breath in the daytime.

If your partner – or any other person – has told you you snore, and you know you are overweight, then you should try to lose the excess. Very often this will cause the snoring problems to stop as well – apart from making you more generally attractive to yourself and other people.

If you don't (or can't) do anything about losing weight, and you continue to snore, then your problem could develop into obstructive sleep apnoea, now known to be the most serious medical risk of all caused by snoring.

SNORING AND OBSTRUCTIVE SLEEP APNOEA (OSA)

This problem affects mainly men – 90 per cent of sufferers are middle-aged men. It is 10 times more common than Parkinson's Disease and 50 times more common than Multiple Sclerosis.

It has been estimated that the average GP practice will have between 10 and 20 cases of OSA among its patients. The presenting symptoms are: a combination of heavy nightly snoring and excessive daytime sleepiness. OSA has been called the 'Pickwickian' syndrome because of Joe, the fat boy in *The Pickwick Papers* who kept falling asleep. The illustration on page 38 of the fat boy, by Harry Furniss, shows a typical sufferer from sleep apnoea – head on one side, complete oblivion as to one's surroundings, and finding it impossible to stay awake.

Although sleep apnoea is less common in young people, the drawing of the fat boy is medically correct in every detail. When sufferers from sleep apnoea go to sleep disorder centres to have their problem assessed, they often drop off to sleep while in the waiting room. They then fall asleep as the doctor talks to them, and they fall asleep before they have finished their own sentences. In fact, they can hardly keep awake. Sufferers from OSA hardly make stimulating companions. Because of their propensity to fall asleep all the time, they may seem stupid – and they are certainly a danger on the roads and when in charge of machinery.

It is estimated that OSA affects between 1 and 4 per cent of the adult population; it is a life-threatening disorder of breathing that occurs only during sleep. Strokes and heart failure can result if the problem is not treated. Many sufferers from this condition are overweight, and around 60 per cent are medically obese.

37

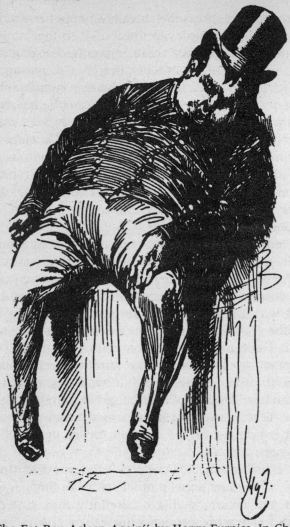

"The Fat Boy Asleep Again" by Harry Furniss. In Charles Dickens, *The Posthumous Papers of the Pickwick Club* (London: The Educational Book Company, 1910).

The condition arises when breathing stops because of the closure of the tissues in the throat, so that no air flows through the sleeper's nose or mouth, despite great efforts to breathe. The sleeper becomes increasingly short of breath until woken up by the *hypoxia* – the brain's reaction to low blood oxygen. Anybody lying next to somebody suffering from sleep apnoea may worry that he or she has actually stopped breathing altogether – then an almighty snort will sound out as the sufferer struggles to breathe again. This may happen hundreds of times during the night, so that the sleeper wakes up exhausted.

'Suffering from sleep apnoea is rather like being at the top of Mount Everest without oxygen,' says sleep expert Dr Christopher Hanning. 'When sufferers are aroused and wake up, their oxygen level goes back to normal, but it falls again the minute they go back to sleep.'

OSA was first described in the medical literature in 1966 and is now very common indeed in the Western world. The back of the throat is the main site of obstruction, and inhalation causes the soft tissues at the back of the throat to collapse. During sleep, the area is narrowed by the combined effects of muscle relaxation, mucous membrane congestion and the tongue being pulled back by gravity. Enlarged tonsils or a bulky tongue can aggravate OSA, but the main cause of the problem is a thick neck – the neck being one of the first places, as we have seen, that fat settles in men.

OSA gets worse with age, as the ageing process produces increasing flabbiness of the soft tissues.

During apnoeas, a number of complicated chemical changes happen. Oxygen levels drop, carbon dioxide levels rise and eventually cause the sleeper to awaken. If he did not wake up, he would probably die in his sleep – which is why apnoeas must always be taken seriously.

It is worth noting that a degree of apnoea is entirely normal. Most people stop breathing in their sleep occasionally. But when it happens five times an hour for 10 seconds or more, then something is definitely wrong and the problem must be addressed.

The obstruction and lack of air put a considerable strain on the heart, and this strain gets worse as the years go by, particularly if the snoring is ignored, as has generally been the case. The lowered blood oxygen that characterizes OSA affects the muscles of the heart and may eventually cause cardiac failure.

Over 70 per cent of patients with OSA will also have high blood-pressure, caused by a rise in blood-pressure during each apnoea. This high blood-pressure continues during waking hours and never returns to normal.

As can be seen, OSA is a complicated condition which adversely affects the workings of many vital organs. But apart from the damage caused to heart muscles and to respiratory function, a sufferer's ordinary, everyday lifestyle will be severely curtailed by OSA.

For one thing, sufferers are extremely dangerous on the roads. They risk falling asleep at the wheel and, until the condition is treated, should never, never drive. If the condition has persisted for a long time, sufferers may not be able to concentrate at work, and may well risk getting the sack. In fact, several patients who were admitted to the sleep disorders centre of a large London hospital were told their jobs were on the line unless they made an effort to stay awake at work. These were all middle-aged executives in the City, with responsible jobs they were no longer able to do properly.

OSA also has a terrible effect on personal and family life. The typical OSA sufferer is a man who always falls asleep in front of the television in the evening; who is always too tired to go out, and who falls asleep when other members of the family are trying to have a conversation with him. He snores loudly in bed, thus annoying everybody even more, and then wakes up exhausted, complaining that he didn't get a wink of sleep all night.

To make matters worse, sufferers from this condition very often wake up with a bad headache, caused, it is believed, by high blood-pressure and the abnormally high levels of carbon dioxide circulating in the system during the frequent apnoeas.

Men who suffer from OSA will not normally have an active sex life. In fact, quite the reverse. They may well suffer from impotence – and even if they don't, their partners are hardly going to be turned on by this overweight, snoring zombie lying beside them.

Nor are these the only complications to arise from OSA. Because the sufferer never gets a good night's sleep – it has been estimated that unless we can sleep in chunks of two minutes at least, we are not refreshed – he is also likely to suffer from severe depression and self-hatred. OSA sufferers will sleep in 30- to 60-second fragments, so that they will wake up feeling like death. In fact, low self-confidence and low self-esteem, coupled with severe depression, are also symptoms of this very serious condition.

Also, because sufferers are always sleepy and tend to be overweight, they cannot find the energy for any exercise. So, as the problem continues, life enters a continual downward spiral, getting less enjoyable all the time and, as the apnoeas continue, ever more dangerous to their health.

No wonder OSA is now taken seriously by doctors working in sleep disorder centres. In fact, the main work of modern sleep laboratories is to assess snoring and see to what extent it is causing sleep disorders and adversely affecting the patient's quality of life.

Not all chronic snorers will develop OSA, but if the snoring is accompanied by all the other factors mentioned, such as overweight and heavy drinking, it is almost inevitable that OSA will eventually result.

In the old days, before OSA was recognized as a proper complaint, such people would have been diagnosed as suffering from insomnia, and the snoring would have been virtually ignored. As such, they would possibly have been prescribed sleeping pills, which would make the problem worse. Drugged sleep is not good sleep – and drugs cannot cure snoring or apnoea.

Now, though, at last, OSA *can* be treated effectively, and previous *joie de vivre* delivered back to sufferers who seemed at times to be enduring a living death.

To sum up, the main symptoms of OSA are:

• loud and incessant snoring

- sudden arousals from sleep, often accompanied by choking
- excessive daytime sleepiness
- awaking from sleep feeling unrefreshed
- constant fatigue and permanent lethargy
- depression that never lifts
- dry throat in the mornings, morning 'muzziness' or headaches
- impotence
- enuresis (bedwetting)
- nocturnal sweating
- changes in personality for the worse.

In addition, a history of nasal injury, asthma or hay fever before the apnoeas become noticeable is common.

ASSESSING THE EXTENT OF THE SNORING

As we have said, snoring is now taken seriously by doctors, because at last there are effective treatments (described in detail in the next two chapters). But in order to get the best possible treatment, it's necessary to take a cool and honest look at your snoring. As you are most probably asleep at the time, you may have to enlist your partner's help – something that he or she will probably only be too glad to offer.

Because snoring is a signal that something is wrong, you should try to overcome any embarrassment about it. After all, it's nothing to be ashamed of, it's simply a medical problem that can be treated.

Here are some questions which will help you to sort

43

out your snoring, so that at last you can do something about it.

Have You Ever Been Told that You Snore?

If the answer to this is 'frequently', then assume that you do – and that people are not just 'ganging up on you'. Few people would go to the trouble of drawing attention to snoring unless it actually were happening.

If the answer to this is 'rarely', then the chances are that your snoring, when and if it occurs, is nothing to worry about, and happens only when you have a cold or other temporary obstruction or infection.

Some people tend to snore when they lie on their backs. This is because this position causes partial blockage of the airways due to the effects of gravity. If your snoring stops when you lie on your side, then you can stop worrying about it. A time-honoured remedy for 'positional snorers' such as these is to sew a tennis or ping-pong ball in the back of their pyjamas, so that every time they roll over onto their backs they are woken up. This simple Pavlovian-type remedy should be tried before embarking on any more complicated treatments.

It is the people who snore in all positions who need to take action. Sleeping on one's side should not cause snoring.

Does Your Snoring Disturb Others?

If the answer to this is 'yes', assume that you are snoring both loudly and frequently. You need to pay attention to it.

Is Your Snoring Getting Worse?

Don't assume that snoring is an inevitable aspect of ageing. It is no more 'natural' to snore when you are old than it is to snore when you are young. If it has become worse over the years, then it definitely needs attention.

Has Your Snoring Ever Caused You to Wake Up, Meant that Your Partner Has Had to Leave the Room to Sleep Somewhere Else, or Has Disturbed the Neighbours?

If the answer to these questions is an emphatic 'yes', then you may well be suffering from sleep apnoea. Even if you are not, you are a serious snorer, especially if you have been aware of daytime sleepiness. Action is needed without delay.

After having read all this, snorers who wonder whether they might be suffering from sleep apnoea should ask themselves these important questions:

- Does it take you a long time to fall asleep at night?
- Do you wake up at night?
- Do you often feel excessively tired on waking up in the morning?
- Do you feel constantly tired during the day?
- Do you tend to fall asleep watching TV, during a lecture, or at work?
- Do you feel in danger of falling asleep at the wheel?
- Do you have difficulty concentrating on your job – more than you used to?

It should be said that daytime sleepiness is not always in itself a sign of sleep apnoea, as there could be other causes. But if the sleepiness is accompanied by loud and terrible snoring at night, then apnoea is extremely likely.

FIRST STEPS TOWARDS TREATMENT

If you believe you may be suffering from OSA, the first thing to do is to go to your doctor and ask for referral to a sleep disorders centre. OSA is not usually something that can be treated simply by self-help measures, although these will be important as well. At the sleep lab, your sleep and your snoring will be monitored precisely, so that you can be given the advice and treatment that are right for your particular case.

Without wishing to be too alarmist, it must be stated that around 3 per cent of sufferers from sleep apnoea will succumb to heart failure unless they get their problem treated as soon as possible.

Quite apart from any health risks, who wants to be a half-asleep zombie all the time?

INTIMATE RELATIONSHIPS

It is only just being recognized that, apart from the toll on physical health, chronic snoring can destroy personal relationships and turn love into hate. Many chronic snorers find themselves banished from bedrooms; repugnance may also set in, levelled against their whole person, not just their snoring. It is almost impossible to overestimate the strain on relationships that long-term snoring can cause.

The situation may perhaps not be too bad in a house

where it's possible to isolate yourself, or where there are plenty of spare bedrooms. But most couples do not have this luxury, and getting out of earshot can be difficult indeed. And if the snorer, or the partner, has to sleep on a sofa feeling he or she is being punished for something over which there seems to be no control, relationships can only suffer and deteriorate.

It is a fact that people dislike you when you start to snore, simply *because* you snore. But even if your nearest and dearest are prepared to put up with the snoring, restorative sleep is not possible – and there will be personality disorders, irritation, an inability to deal with stress, and chronic bad temper. In addition to this, new research into the subject is showing that spouses often use snoring as an *excuse* to turn their partners out of the bedroom, or to sleep separately.

Dr John Stradling, who has studied snoring and its effects, says:

> *We frequently get people coming to the sleep laboratory complaining that their spouse snores all night long. Yet when the snoring is objectively measured, it lasts for perhaps 10 minutes. But because the snorer is asleep at the time, it's impossible to argue.*
>
> *We do find, though, that marital harmony is often restored when the snorer decides to do something positive about the snoring. It is the ability to please the partner which seems to count higher than actually stopping snoring.*
>
> *When partners complain, snoring is very often grossly over-reported.*

Dr Stradling says that in almost all these cases, alcohol

is involved. A very common scenario is that the husband drinks too much at the pub, at parties or other functions, and then comes home drunk. Because of this, he snores. But because most people are extremely reluctant to admit that they have drunk too much, or that they do so on a regular basis, a wife's complaints about the drinking are not likely to have an effect. If, however, she complains about his loud snoring, and threatens to go to another bedroom, or turns him out of the marital bed, then eventually the snoring problem might be addressed.

It is well known that alcohol and overeating are the most likely causes of chronic snoring. If people can reduce their alcohol intake – and this is not easy, as any heavy drinker knows – then the snoring is likely to ease up.

As Dr Stradling says, the issues around snoring and marital harmony are extremely complex and are only just beginning to be addressed. After 15 or 20 years of marriage, very many women long for the deep peace of the single – or at least, the separate – bed, but very often, husbands are reluctant either to go to the spare room, or to sleep alone in the marital bed.

There is some evidence to suggest that men like sleeping with women more than women like sleeping with men. (I'm using 'sleeping' here in its literal sense, not as a euphemism for sex.) A woman's preference for sleeping alone also intensifies with age, and therefore it is almost always the wife who first suggests separate beds or separate rooms.

As most men do eventually begin to snore after middle age, and especially if they gain fat around the upper part of the body (as the majority do after the age of 40), then complaints of snoring can be a potent weapon in the campaign for separate rooms.

All this is not to say that snoring is not a serious problem, or that the health risks connected with it have been exaggerated. But very often, a partner's assessment of snoring will be extremely subjective, especially if – as is common in long-term relationships – a substantial degree of marital disharmony already exists.

One of the reasons men may be so willing to have their snoring levels recorded, and to try patent cures and inventions to stop the noise, is that at all costs they would like to preserve the marital status quo and continue to sleep with their wives.

There is now a great deal of evidence to support the idea that men are far more traumatized than women by divorce, and several recent studies have shown that women are, on the whole, happier than men to live alone. There seems little doubt that the great majority of snorers are men, but sleep experts are now saying that we need to take with a pinch of salt some wives' claims that they never sleep a wink all night because of their husbands' loud snoring.

Sleep scientists are now saying that more research is needed into the question of marriage, long-term relationships and snoring. It appears, from some preliminary studies, that wives complain of their husbands' snoring when they start to grow tired of them and irritated by them. A new partner who snored just as much would probably not call forth the same amount of irritation.

Also, over the years, it can become difficult to enjoy sleeping with anybody who has come to irritate you greatly, so it is possible that even light snores will wake you up.

None of this, however, means that snoring is normal, or that it should be ignored. It's just that the connection between snoring and the actual relationship between the bedpartners can make an enormous difference to the way in which the snoring is perceived and whether it is considered a terrible nuisance, a mild irritation, or even an endearing habit.

CHAPTER THREE

Treating the Problem

At the very least, snoring is always a nuisance. If you are told you snore – and you have reason to believe what you are told – then you should take action sooner rather than later.

Although severe cases of 'heroic' snoring may need careful investigation in a sleep laboratory, in many instances snoring can be prevented by a few simple home measures.

If you snore most nights, even though this may not be all that loud or bad enough to wake the neighbours, start off by taking an objective look at your sleeping positions. Snoring is almost always made worse, and may in fact be caused, by sleeping on your back.

You may have to train yourself to sleep on your side. This can be done using a special pillow, or by using ordinary pillows or bolsters to make sure you stay on your side. The trick of sewing a tennis ball into the pocket of your pyjamas or T-shirt is an old remedy that often works.

Anything that trains you to sleep on your side will tend to alleviate the problem, although it may not stop the snoring altogether. But sleeping on your back is the very worst position for anyone who snores – or who may potentially snore.

NASAL CONGESTION

This often causes snoring. If it's temporary, then it's nothing to worry about. But as the simple act of lying down in itself causes a degree of congestion, people who suffer in this way should try to sleep with their head and shoulders raised. This prevents the congestion, and may even clear up the problem of snoring.

The British Sleep Society's booklet *Snoring and What to Do About It* recommends using a wedge of foam under the bottom sheet. It should measure about 30 in/75 cm long, 26 in/65 cm wide and 8 in/20 cm high. It can be made from a block of foam 4 in/10 cm high sliced diagonally, with one section turned round. People who have tried this say that it does work – but the foam is expensive to buy.

Note: almost all anti-snoring devices and treatments tend to make the sufferer less sexually alluring, and for this reason people are often embarrassed to use them. But faced with a choice, it's always better to try to stop the snoring, or get to the bottom of the problem, than to worry about whether you are the world's sexiest person. The chances are that nobody will fancy you for very long if you keep him or her awake all night with your snoring.

It's a sad fact that all the myriad books on sexual positions and how to have a good sex life never mention snoring as a possible turn-off – or even how common it is. People are often shocked and surprised when they get married, or live permanently with a partner, to discover that the love of their life snores. It's something they are not prepared for.

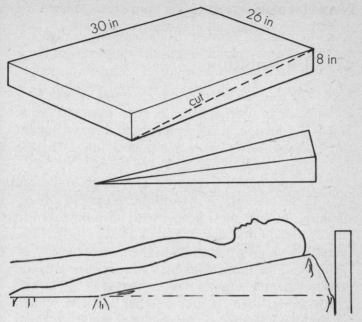

A foam wedge under the bottom sheet can help prevent snoring.

CHANGES IN LIFESTYLE

There are a few lifestyle changes which can often make the difference between silent nights and loud snoring. One is not to drink alcohol late at night. Another is to make sure you eat early in the evening whenever possible. Stop smoking if you possibly can. Apart from all the other reasons why smoking is a bad idea, cigarette smoke is an irritant and causes inflammation and increased mucus production in the throat. You

53

know how often smokers suffer from excess phlegm – a well-known congestant and cause of snoring.

Give Up Smoking

According to some snoring experts, smoking can be a major cause of snoring because, apart from increasing mucus production, it causes lung and throat irritation and increased secretions from bronchial tubes. There is also reduced oxygen uptake by the lungs.

For most people it is relatively easy to eat and drink early in the evenings. It may not be so easy to give up smoking. In fact, most people who have managed to give up reckon that stopping smoking was the hardest thing they've ever had to do in their whole lives.

However, for those who just can't seem to give up, who feel that life without nicotine would simply not be worth living, there is now another solution which, while still not being good for you, does much less harm than smoking. This is to chew nicotine gum when the craving strikes.

Nicotine gum was originally developed for submariners who just could not smoke, but who went round the bend without their nicotine fix. The gum delivers an acceptable amount of nicotine, but without the harmful effects that smoking brings. It doesn't affect the lungs, nor irritate the throat.

Limit Alcohol

Alcohol is also a potent cause of snoring. In fact, very many people are 'alcohol snorers' – snoring only when they've had too much to drink. That's okay if you are an occasional drinker, indulging only once in a while.

But if you are a regular or heavy drinker, you may find that snoring is a nightly problem. One recent study in the US showed that even middle-aged men who snored rarely, always did so after drinking a lot of alcohol. Alcohol also produces sleep apnoeas – a serious health problem for chronic heavy drinkers.

Those who already know they have a snoring problem should make sure they never have an alcoholic nightcap just before bed and should watch their alcohol consumption very carefully. Those who have already had sleep apnoea diagnosed, or who are extremely heavy snorers, should do their utmost to cut their alcohol consumption.

As we know, for many people this is easier said than done. As is well known by organizations such as Alcoholics Anonymous (AA), drink-related problems thrive on denial. How many people do you know who admit they drink too much, too often? Doctors in general practice and in sleep laboratories are often in absolute despair over patients who can't seem to stop drinking. The patients are given good advice on cutting down their drinking, yet they can't seem to follow it, even though their health is being ruined in the process.

The reason? They are addicted – and can no longer choose whether to drink or not. Most people who drink heavily and regularly find it impossible to cut down. They will also say they enjoy drinking, will resent being told how much they ought to drink and will probably have no real idea how much they are consuming. They may also vehemently deny that they snore.

It's a very difficult problem, because alcohol is known to be insidiously addictive and extremely difficult to control. It is also unlikely that anybody with a drinking problem who is also a heavy snorer will be able to give up by sheer willpower. Anybody who has a serious snoring problem, or who has developed sleep apnoea and who also drinks, may find it worthwhile to join a group such as AA, which has a better record for helping people with alcohol problems than any other organization.

The problem is, the drinker – or the snorer – has to find within him- or herself the motivation to join a group to help cut down or abstain completely from drinking. It's no use the doctor or partner advising it – such advice will only be rejected. And, over the years, alcohol has become such a friend.

It's easy to say 'make a few simple lifestyle changes' – but the trouble is that all the habits which cause or exacerbate snoring – smoking, drinking, overeating – are potent addictions and by no means easy to control or overcome. However – it *can* be done – and don't be afraid to enlist help if you find the going tough on your own. There are many organizations to help people stop smoking, to overcome drinking problems and to cope with overeating.

The Question of Self-esteem

Because snoring is often, erroneously, associated with character and personality defects, when in fact it is a physical dysfunction, people who know they snore often suffer from very low self-esteem. They drink too much, they smoke too much, they eat too much and nobody likes them because they snore. In addition, they may keep falling asleep in the daytime.

If you are a loud snorer, nobody wants to sleep with you. Nobody even wants to sleep in the same room as you. In severe cases, nobody even wants to sleep in the same house. Therefore, you can feel extremely excluded, isolated and unloved.

If at the same time you can't seem to cut down your alcohol or cigarette consumption, you are going to feel even worse about yourself – and may wonder whether life is worth living. And if your job and/or relationship is at risk because of your snoring/sleepiness, then you get a whole spectrum of problems which are not easy to sort out.

The thing is to take problems one at a time. It is not possible to give up smoking, drinking and overeating all at once. So take it bit by bit: decide what you are going to tackle first and stick with it until you have made definite progress. Then move on to the next thing. With each lifestyle problem that you overcome, your self-esteem and self-confidence will grow – and there will be the bonus that you are not snoring so much and have more energy during the daytime as well.

All snorers feel bad about themselves, because nobody likes to be thought of as a snorer. And often, by the time snoring has become a real problem, bad habits have become ingrained to the extent that they are difficult to overcome. Difficult they may be, but never impossible.

Losing Weight

Many snorers are overweight. Overweight, as we have seen, causes snoring, particularly in men. When women put on weight, it tends to gather round their hips and thighs – hence the runaway success of hip-and-thigh diet books – but men tend to accumulate flab around the upper part of the body, especially around the neck.

Losing weight, like stopping smoking and cutting down drinking, is always easier said than done, but it is essential if you are serious about wanting to stop snoring. Mostly, people get used to eating a certain amount over the years and feel horribly deprived when they have to cut down.

I have no easy solutions to offer – obviously anybody can write out a diet that will be highly effective so long as people manage to stick to it. The trouble with diets is that people can't stick to them – not that they don't work, as has been alleged. So whenever weight is lost, it tends to go back on again.

Determination can soon be overcome by the smell and taste of a really delicious meal, and very often seriously overweight people need a major health jolt to give them the motivation to cut down on their eating. The thing to do is enlist the help of others. Get your partner to help you to stick to your diet, get a diet sheet from the doctor, or spend a week at a health farm.

Although health farms are expensive, you will be absolutely guaranteed to lose weight, as food is just not available, and losses of a stone in a week are not uncommon. Also, as health farms are so very expensive, and you will tend to feel so good when you come away, there will be a greater reluctance to start putting weight back on straight away.

Good health farms nowadays teach their guests how to re-educate their palates so that the weight will not be put back on again. I can't pretend that eating lettuce leaves and unbuttered bread is as delicious as hot toast dripping with butter, which seems to satisfy the soul as well as the body, but in time you will get used to it – and even enjoy the subtler taste sensations that come from eating fresh, unprocessed foods.

You should also try cutting down on dairy products, as these are now known to be allergy-producing in many people, and also mucus-forming. As yet there have been no clinical trials on the possible connection between dairy foods and snoring, but if you feel permanently blocked-up and sinusy, it may be worth trying to go vegan for a time, to see whether avoiding eating animal fats makes a difference.

POSITIVE ANTI-SNORING TREATMENTS

Yoga

One of the best ways of treating snoring is to learn to breathe through the nose. You will certainly learn to do this at a good yoga class.

In fact, around 20 minutes at the beginning of each class will be spent in *pranayama* – correct breathing techniques. The pranayama exercises consist of deep abdominal breathing and alternate nostril breathing.

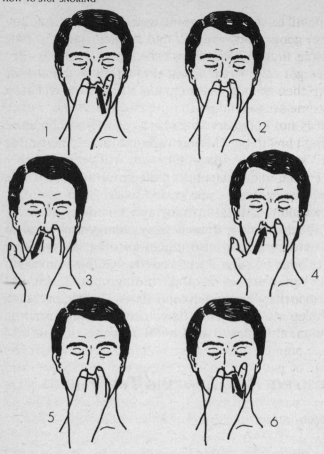

Correct breathing exercise: 1. Holding your right nostril closed with your thumb, breathe in through your left nostril. 2. Hold in the breath while you close both nostrils. 3. Keeping the left nostril closed with your ring and little finger, breathe out through your right nostril. 4. Breathe in through the right nostril. 5. Hold in the breath while you close both nostrils. 6. Keeping your right nostril closed with your thumb, breathe out through your left nostril.

You will be shown exactly how to do this and, like any other good habit, you will find it takes practice. Some people find the breathing exercises difficult, as they have got used to breathing through their mouths, or with their mouths open. But with practise it will soon become second-nature.

It is not necessary to go to a yoga class to practise correct breathing. This can easily be done at home (see the illustration on page 60).

If you find alternate nostril breathing a problem, this may be because you have some obstruction or congestion which merits further investigation or treatment. You may well find, however, that yoga sessions cure your breathing problems. They will also have other benefits, such as encouraging you not to eat heavy meals late at night, not drinking, and learning to relax so that your sleep is more refreshing without being so deep and drug-like that you start to snore again.

Yoga, although so ancient, is becoming a more and more popular form of exercise. This is because it can be done by people of any age and at any fitness level, and the benefits are quickly appreciated. Yoga exercises every part of the body in turn, and also helps to aid digestion and breathing in everyday life.

Nasal Decongestants

If the problem seems to be chronic nasal congestion, then decongestants may be able to help. There are two kinds available – those sold over the counter and those on prescription. It's best, according to sleep expert Dr

Christopher Hanning, to go for the ones on prescription, as the over-the-counter remedies can set up irritations in the nose and should be used only occasionally.

You can also get special anti-snoring sprays. These are supposed to keep the airways open, but apparently they only work for a short time and, as snoring is usually a chronic problem, a more permanent remedy is needed. In any case, anti-snoring sprays do not cure the problem, as the airways close up again as soon as you stop using the spray.

The Bedroom

If you snore, it is important to pay careful attention to the bedroom, bearing in mind that snoring is rarely a problem that will go away of its own accord. As well as making sure your sleeping position is the one least likely to cause snoring, you should also ensure that your bedroom gives you optimum sleeping conditions. The ideal temperature for a bedroom is cool – 64–66°F/18–19°C, so that you don't feel hot and stuffy in bed. A firm mattress – a rubber *Dunlopillo* is a good idea as it is both firm and eliminates allergy problems coming from house dust mites – and a pillow that keeps your neck straight, are both worthwhile investments.

Patent Remedies

Ever since time began, inventive minds have been trying to work out an anti-snoring cure that works.

Most of the old-time ones didn't have much of an effect, largely because the mechanism of snoring was poorly understood.

But modern patent remedies, which have often been subjected to stringent clinical trials, really can make a difference. And it is always worth trying the small, cheap, easy remedies before embarking on complicated tests at sleeping laboratories and the like.

One of the most successful recent anti-snoring inventions is the *Nozovent*, a small plastic device for dilating the nostrils. It was invented in Sweden and has undergone a number of clinical trials.

The ideal customer for the *Nozovent*, which is now available at most chemists', is somebody who is not overweight, elderly or given to over-indulgence in food or drink, but who snores because of a nasal problem. Young, slim, healthy people who snore at night will very often have something slightly anatomically wrong with their noses, such as a deviated septum, which makes them snore. For them a device such as the *Nozovent* can effectively overcome their snoring.

The *Nozovent* works like this. If you pull your nostrils open and breathe, you will find that the air moves freely and easily and you have no desire to open your mouth. The *Nozovent* does in your sleep what you are doing for yourself with your fingers – it keeps your nostrils wide apart.

The *Nozovent* was invented and developed by a Swedish ENT surgeon, Dr Bjorn Petruson, of the University Hospital of Göteborg. The first clinical trial on the device was carried out in 1988 on 50 patients who were all chronic snorers. 34 were men and 16 were

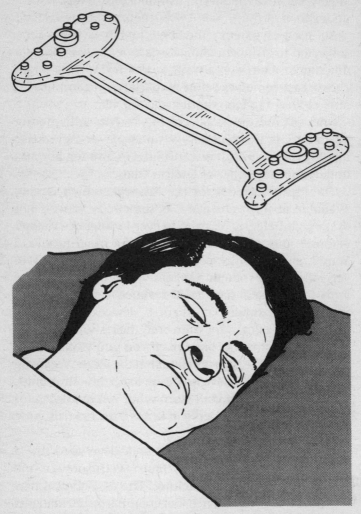

The *Nozovent*

women; most were aged between 40 and 50. A deviated nasal septum was found in eight of the patients, and three were recommended to have special nasal surgery (this will be discussed further in Chapter 4). Eight patients had a narrowed nasal valve.

For the study, the patients were asked to use the dilator every second night for about four weeks, and then report back. They were asked to record their snoring and periods of being awake during the night – possibly with the help of a partner – and also note whether they were tired or had a dry mouth in the morning. (Breathing through the mouth often produces a dry mouth and can be a sign that you've been snoring during the night). The patients were also asked to record whether they had noticed any difference in the quality of sleep when using the nasal dilator.

They were also asked other questions about the device, such as whether it fell out easily and whether it was - generally comfortable and aesthetically acceptable to use.

Results showed that of the initial 50 patients, 44 noticed a dramatic difference in the quality of their sleep when using the device. 26 patients were extremely heavy snorers: for 23 of them, the snoring decreased considerably with the device in place.

About 50 per cent of the patients felt less tired when sleeping with a dilated nose. 80 per cent noted less dryness in their mouths in the morning, indicating that they had not breathed through the mouth, and 33 per cent remarked that the dryness disappeared altogether when using the device.

On the whole, the men coped quite well with the

dilator, but women disliked using it, not because it was in any way uncomfortable, but because they felt it made them look ugly while asleep.

In another study, reported in the *Archives of Otolaryngology – Head and Neck Surgery* (April, 1990) 10 patients used the *Nozovent* every other night, and their partners were asked to record their snoring levels using an agreed scoring system. The patients – eight men and two women aged between 25 and 50 – had all been snoring regularly for more than eight years.

The scoring was as follows: 0 = no snoring; 1 = slight snoring; 2 = moderate snoring; 3 = severe snoring. In total, 50 nights with and 50 nights without the device were recorded.

The results showed that for the nights when the device was used, the total snoring score was 45 points, and that for the nights without it, the score went up to 90 points. This represented an overall decrease from moderate to slight snoring.

When the device was used, on 14 out of 50 nights the snorers' partners heard no snoring at all, compared to one night out of 50 when the device was not used. Severe snoring was noted on 12 nights when the dilator was not used, compared to one night when it was used.

When the nasal valve is dilated with the help of the device, the airflow through the nose is increased to greater than normal. It is thought that resulting drop in pressure needed to breathe while unconscious means that the palate and soft tissues of the throat do not start vibrating.

Most ENT surgeons and sleep specialists are in favour of the *Nozovent*, which they feel has replaced other

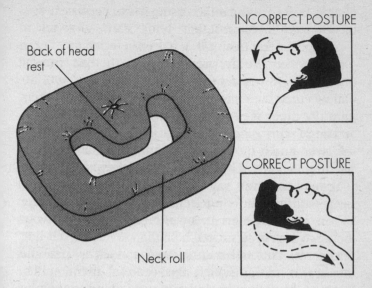

INCORRECT POSTURE

CORRECT POSTURE

Back of head
rest

Neck roll

The *Snorestop* pillow

devices to keep the nasal passages dilated. They recommend that it should be tried before the snorer resorts – or is recommended – for nasal surgery or a CPAP unit.

Although the *Nozovent* can certainly work, it should not be used if you suffer from any nasal congestion. If you have a cold, nasal polyps or suffer from allergies such as hay fever or allergic rhinitis that can give you a blocked-up nose, you will have to have these attended to before expecting the device to work.

The Snorestop

This is a special pillow designed to enable the snorer to sleep without obstructing the air passages.

67

The pillow, which is made from polyester, was developed in conjunction with ENT surgeons at Oldham General Hospital. It has been tested on only 14 patients, but the average reduction in their snoring levels was 78 per cent. Some patients found that the pillow cured their snoring problems absolutely; others, that the noise was at least considerably reduced.

The *Snorestop* pillow is much more expensive than the *Nozovent*, and is most useful for snorers whose problem seems to be caused by their incorrect sleeping positions. The manufacturers say that the pillow can also be of help to those suffering from sleep apnoea, although when apnoea seems to be the problem it is always better to seek professional help than to rely on self-help measures. This is because sleep apnoea is a serious medical condition which needs careful attention. The surgeon or sleep specialist may well recommend a special pillow, although it is likely that a more holistic approach will be needed to cure this very serious snoring problem.

Note: There are a number of other patent anti-snoring devices on the market, such as special wrist devices which wake you up when you snore. Most ENT and sleep specialists do not recommend these, however. The two devices described above are the only ones which have actually been subjected to trials and been found to work for a majority of volunteers.

CHAPTER FOUR

Medical and Surgical Treatments for Snoring

In many cases, the home remedies and treatments outlined in Chapter 3 will be enough to prevent snoring, or at least to turn it from a major nuisance into simply a mild annoyance.

Some snoring experts suggest that self-help remedies – particularly the lifestyle changes – should be tried for around three months to see if they work. If the snoring is just as bad in spite of all your efforts to cut down on your drinking, smoking and overeating, then more drastic measures may need to be taken.

Of all self-help remedies, that of losing weight will be by far the most beneficial to the snorer. Most doctors and ENT surgeons now agree that this should take top priority in any serious stop-snoring regime.

It is only when really loud, unacceptable snoring persists after weight loss, or if, once your ideal weight has been achieved, this has not made an appreciable difference to snoring levels, that the medical and surgical remedies described here should be tried.

But however bad, however loud, never imagine that your snoring problem cannot be helped. It can – it's just a matter of finding the right remedy for you. This may take time, especially if you have been snoring loudly for many years.

Before taking your problem to the doctor, it's most important to monitor your snoring with a tape recorder set near your bed, so that you can know for sure whether the treatments you are trying are really making any difference.

A tape recorder will give you an accurate guide as to the efficacy of self-help methods. If they don't seem to be affecting the problem to any great extent, don't despair. There are now very many medical treatments on offer which can either cure or completely prevent snoring, so that you and all around you can get a decent night's sleep. Don't forget – you owe it both to yourself and to others to try to stop snoring.

Of course, it can seem like adding insult to injury to stop smoking, cut down on alcohol and all your favourite foods, to wear a nasal dilator, learn to sleep on your side, sew an uncomfortable tennis ball into your pyjamas or make a foam wedge – in other words, to have to make serious attempts to cure your snoring problem when the only result is that you are snoring as loudly as before.

All that deprivation – and for no result!

But at least by trying all the home remedies and lifestyle changes you are taking the problem seriously – and you will certainly feel better and more alert in the daytime for eating more healthily and drinking less.

SLEEP LABORATORIES AND SLEEP DISORDERS CENTRES

If in spite of everything you continue to snore

unacceptably loudly, the next step will be to request referral to a sleep laboratory.

In the US, sleep laboratories and sleep disorders centres have become extremely big business, possibly because snoring and sleep apnoea are particularly big problems there. Sleep clinics were first set up by psychiatrist Dr William Dement, who first drew attention to the medical problems that could be caused by insomnia, sleep apnoea and snoring. Dr Dement now believes that sleep deprivation – for whatever reason – is a major cause of ill-health, injury and depression. Dr Dement is now working on trying to establish definite links between sleep disorders and physical problems.

All regular snorers, as well as their partners and those within hearing, are likely to be deprived of sleep over a long period of time, says Dr Dement, and this can lead to a host of other problems, mental, physical and emotional. And as the only real way to assess snoring and its effect on sleep and oxygen levels is by assessment in a sleep laboratory, Dr Dement is now calling for the establishment of more sleep disorder centres and for this problem to be taken seriously by the American government.

In the UK, there are now about 25 medically-supervised sleep disorder centres, several of which are attached to large teaching hospitals. The existence and proliferation of sleep laboratories over the past 10 years is a sure sign that sleep problems and snoring are at last being taken seriously and may need careful medical assessment and attention. They are a potent indication that the days when snoring was considered merely a minor complaint are well and truly over.

Allen Davey, founder of the British Snoring and Sleep Apnoea Association and a heavy snorer himself, believes that doctors and surgeons running sleep labs are the unsung heroes of our time – helping people to overcome a problem that previously few dared even mention.

It's a fact that many spouses are extremely nervous of telling their partners that they snore – and put up with the row without saying anything, often for years on end, for fear of getting an earful of denials and accusations if they do. But it's hardly conducive to a loving relationship, and the non-snoring partner risks going without sleep, thus intensifying the problems of sleep deprivation described by Dr Dement.

Admittedly, it may seem rather alarming to be admitted to a sleep laboratory for something that sounds so insignificant as snoring and be wired up to a machine which people are monitoring closely in the next room. Imagine – strangers are not only going to hear you snore, they are also going to be assessing the levels, something you would probably rather keep to yourself. Also, to some people, it seems like taking a lot of trouble and NHS time and money when people are dying of more serious diseases.

But remember – sleep disorders centres exist to help with exactly the problem you have. They will certainly take your snoring problem seriously, even if nobody else does, because they know from research of the harm it can cause, both to the snorer and anyone else who has to listen to the snoring.

So what are sleep laboratories like? The answer is: far

less intimidating than they seem. Mostly, they consist of two small adjoining rooms, one where you as the patient will sleep, the other where the technician will sit and monitor your sleep, oxygen and snoring levels. The rooms for sleeping are made as comfortable as possible, and all you see of the machine(s) is a series of wires passing through to the next room.

Many patients, on entering a sleep laboratory, wonder how on earth they will sleep, in this strange room and wired up to sophisticated machinery. There may also be embarrassment about snoring – it all seems so out of their control, and possibly not the image they would like to present. But admitting the problem is half the battle. If you have these worries about a sleep lab, try to bear in mind that the doctors and technicians there hear people snoring every night. That's what they are there for, so it's no big deal to them. They won't laugh, make jokes or say you are a 'champion snorer'; they will take your complaint seriously and view your snoring as a sign of a possibly serious medical condition. They will even *like* your snoring – it will show up dramatically on their machines and they will be very pleased for you to try their arsenal of stop-snoring treatments.

Even if your snoring is not found to be all that serious, it will be treated as a genuine condition and you will be given sympathetic help on how best to deal with it.

But usually, by the time your snoring has become serious enough to merit investigation at a sleep laboratory, it will probably be badly affecting your life anyway.

Initially you will be referred to the laboratory by your

doctor and admitted for an initial consultation. In some sleep centres, your spouse will be invited along as well, as for most couples snoring is very much a joint problem. Most labs recommend that couples should try to sort out the snoring problem together.

The doctor in charge will first take a detailed case history, asking when the snoring first started and how bad it seems to be. He or she will also ask questions about alcohol and food intake. Try to answer all these questions honestly – if you know you drink too much in the evenings, for example, say so. Evasive answers won't help to cure the problem.

If you are male – and the great majority of serious snorers admitted to sleep labs are – one of the most important questions the doctor will ask you is your collar size. He or she will also want to know whether you have tried any patent anti-snoring remedies, or tried to change your eating and drinking habits lately.

Then, if he or she is satisfied that you have a problem the laboratory can address, you will be admitted for up to three nights. The first will be to get you used to the place, the second to record the problem and the third, if necessary, to try out any treatments considered suitable for your problem.

Sometimes, people do find they can't sleep on the first night as it all seems so strange. Mostly the rooms where you sleep – always on your own – are small and cell-like, with little in the way of distractions. Most people find that by the third night they are sleeping extremely peacefully, and often the quality of sleep in the lab will be the best they've enjoyed for years.

In the morning, you will be shown the readings on

the machines, and they will be interpreted to you. The machines record not only your snore levels, but your blood-oxygen level and heart-rate. There will be no blood tests or injections or any type of invasive treatment. Nothing will hurt.

Mostly, the machines will be recording shallow obstructive breathing and, when apnoeas occur, those times when there is no breathing at all.

Then, when the doctor is satisfied that enough information is known about your snoring, he or she will discuss with you the treatments on offer – and their implications. If you are overweight, you will almost certainly be advised to lose weight before either committing yourself to an operation or a lifetime on a CPAP machine.

If the machines show up the sleep apnoea as being really bad, however, the doctor may decide to put you on a machine straight away. All snorers are different, which is why the only accurate way of assessing your particular problem is to spend a night or two in a sleep disorders centre.

CPAP Units

If you suffer from sleep apnoea, as do many of the people who are referred to sleep laboratories, then you will most probably be recommended a CPAP unit. These deliver air during the night through a tightly-fitting but comfortable mask, and they have such an immediate and dramatic effect that OSA sufferers often feel completely different people after just one night on the machine.

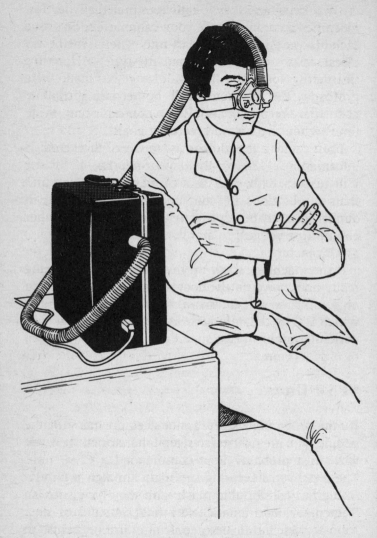

A CPAP unit in place

It then becomes clear to sufferers that their daytime sleepiness, mood swings, depression, tiredness and lack of concentration are all caused by what their body does at night, rather than from stress at work, getting old, or the possibility that middle-age has made them crotchety and bad-tempered. Something springs to life – and the contrast is often remarkable and swift.

CPAP units, which are becoming smaller and more sophisticated all the time, were first developed in Australia in 1981 by Dr Colin Sullivan, of Sydney University. The idea is that airway collapse – which causes heavy snoring and apnoea – is prevented by pumping continuous pressure through the night when the patient is asleep.

The pump generates enough pressure to hold the tissues apart – the amount of pressure depends on each individual and the amount of collapse. CPAP units have to be carefully fitted and evaluated, which is why they are available only through hospitals and are not on general sale.

They are quite expensive, costing several hundred pounds, but in some hospitals they may be available on loan and, in rare cases in the UK, available on the NHS. Newmarket General Hospital, for instance, has a budget to supply CPAP units to sleep apnoea sufferers, although in most other hospital units the patient would have to find the money.

If a CPAP unit seems to be the best treatment for you, you may well be put in touch with somebody who has been using one for some time. A number of sleep laboratories have these 'pairing' arrangements, as talking to someone who has experienced using a CPAP unit can help you considerably with the nervousness and reluctance you may have about using one yourself.

Advantages and Disadvantages of CPAP Units

The main advantages of CPAP units is that they do away with the need for nasal or throat surgery, and they make an astonishing difference to the quality of sleep – and therefore, energy levels in the daytime.

There are, however, several disadvantages to the units, the major one being that they have to be used for as long as the apnoeas are likely to persist – that is, for the rest of the patient's life.

There is also a potent sexual turn-off effect. The sleeper has to have a big mask on his nose, which is connected by a tube to the unit that supplies the pressure. CPAPs therefore make extremely effective contraceptives, as few people are likely to be turned on by a man in a CPAP unit.

Also, they are not a cure, but only a treatment. If ever you stop using the unit, the snoring and apnoea problems are likely to return. They provide symptomatic relief – management of the problem, you might say – but do not remove it. The tissues in the throat will still be in partial collapse, and no amount of air going through at night will make much difference to that.

Another disadvantage is that they make a noise rather like a fan heater, and this may disturb some partners. However, most partners maintain that the noise of the CPAP unit is nothing compared to what they've had to put up with for years with the snoring.

One solution to the noise problem may be to have the unit in another room. This would mean having an enormously long tube though, and so far technology has not provided a happy solution to this hurdle.

The mask has to be completely airtight, otherwise it won't work, and some patients find it uncomfortable, or simply never get used to it. The masks used to be made of rubber, which went hard and absorbed smells after a time, but the newest ones are made of silicone, an inert material that is very soft and pliable and does not pick up smells, grime or fluff either from the sleeper or the bed or bedroom.

Because CPAPs are expensive, bulky and, for some patients, difficult to use, they tend to be reserved for serious OSA sufferers only. 'They work on everybody without exception,' says sleep specialist Dr Christopher Hanning:

> There are a variety of ways of delivering the air, and we try to make the unit as acceptable as possible to the patient.
>
> There are no long-term side effects, no hazards, and it is one of the most gratifying treatments in existence. The family are usually extremely grateful as they no longer have to put up with a snoring, sleepy zombie.
>
> We find that, when fitted with the units, patients usually sleep like logs for the first time in years. They say they can't remember when they woke up and felt so good.

Most of the CPAP and BiPAP units (the BiPAP is a refinement on the original model which can reduce air

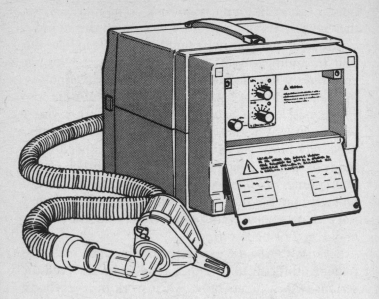

The BiPAP unit

pressure for the exhalation phase and which is recommended for some OSA sufferers) are American, although there is now one British company, SiPlan, which has developed a range of CPAP units in conjunction with Newmarket General Hospital.

SiPlan makes a suitcase model which can also be taken for visits to hotels and when staying in other people's homes.

One of the factors people often don't appreciate enough about snoring is that social life can be extremely curtailed. Sufferers can be extremely reluctant to stay in other people's homes, it can be difficult for them to go on holiday, and as the snoring

80

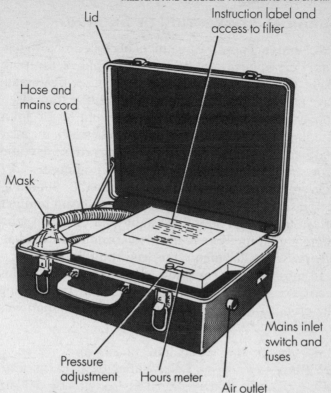

Lid

Instruction label and
access to filter

Hose and
mains cord

Mask

Pressure
adjustment

Hours meter

Air outlet

Mains inlet
switch and
fuses

The suitcase-model CPAP unit

gets worse they are increasingly confined to their own
homes – and even there, they are often not made to feel
very welcome. No wonder the poor snorer feels like,
and is treated as, a social outcast.

The CPAP units can effectively cancel out all
problems connected with severe snoring – but the units
themselves are quite a nuisance to use, set up and carry
around.

81

SURGICAL CORRECTION OF SNORING

CPAP units are now the treatment of choice for sufferers from sleep apnoea, and the worse the apnoea, the more likely the unit is to succeed where other treatments have failed. But not all heavy snorers suffer from sleep apnoea. In the Oxford study carried out by Dr John Stradling, referred to earlier, 850 men between the ages of 35 and 65 snored heavily enough to cause daytime drowsiness but were not sufferers from apnoea.

Even so, the snoring was, as considered Dr Stradling, serious enough to be the cause of a significant number of car crashes. Dr Stradling established that men who snore are six times more likely to crash their cars than otherwise similar men who sleep soundly at night.

In most of the cases studied by Dr Stradling and his team, excess tissue at the back of the throat was causing the problem. In these cases, the only real solution was to excise this tissue.

UPPP

The operation, which by all accounts is far worse to pronounce than to perform, is known as *uvulopalatopharyngoplasty*, or UPPP. It can be extremely successful for heavy snorers who do not suffer from sleep apnoea. Again, assessment would be needed in a sleep laboratory to determine whether this operation would be successful, as it does not work for OSA.

As with CPAP units, UPPP should be considered only after careful evaluation and after self-help remedies and lifestyle adjustments have been tried. As with using a

CPAP unit, UPPP is a drastic measure and should be considered a last resort; and unlike using a CPAP, UPPP is not reversible!

In the UK, ENT surgeons are quite reluctant to perform UPPP, except as a final measure when all else has failed. In the US, however, it is performed commonly to cure snoring problems. Unlike the CPAP, UPPP is actually a cure, not just a treatment. If the operation is successful, you will snore no more – guaranteed.

The operation was developed especially as a cure for snoring by the Japanese. Early versions of UPPP were carried out as long ago as 1952, but it was not until 1980 that it was perfected in its present form. Basically, the operation consists of removing the uvula, tonsils (if any) and part of the soft palate. This has the effect of enlarging the passages and keeping the airways open when the patient is asleep.

The operation is quite easy to perform, but like all throat operations it is delicate and needs skill. It consists of opening up the air passages by widening and opening the back of the throat. Dr Christopher Hanning likens the result to having a bell with no clapper – and we all know how impossible it is for a bell to ring once its clapper has gone.

Most doctors in the UK screen patients very carefully indeed before recommending UPPP, as the operation can have adverse side-effects, such as causing the patient to regurgitate food and drink through the nose afterwards. Although this is described as a possibly permanent hazard, in fact most patients find that this problem clears up after a few weeks.

It's also essential to screen patients carefully for this operation because, after they've had it, the CPAP unit no longer works. Therefore, it should be carried out only on patients who do not need the CPAP.

Most people would probably rather undergo a one-off operation which has a reasonable chance of success than have to wear a CPAP in bed for the rest of their lives – but it's all a matter of suitability and assessing each patient's type of snoring and the problems associated with it.

Most surgeons now feel that UPPP has stood the test of time successfully and that few complications now result, as long as the operation is carried out by a competent surgeon. ENT surgeon Dr Michael Gleeson of Guy's Hospital, London, has now carried out very many UPPP operations. He recently followed up 22 patients with 'socially unacceptable' snoring who were treated by UPPP between January 1987 and December 1990. There were 20 males and two females altogether. The age range of patients was 21 to 68, proving that you do not have to be a fat old man to be a heavy snorer.

The patients had snored heavily for 11 years on average and other methods to try to stop the noise had not worked. Before the operation was carried out, the patients' bedpartners were asked to assess the snoring on a scale from one to four – that is, from no snoring to intolerable snoring. Before the operation, every single patient had scored four.

Also before the operation, each patient had attempted to lose weight to try to reduce snoring levels in this way. Some had failed to lose weight whereas others, while managing to get their weight down to normal, still snored as loudly as before. All patients had excess soft tissue and elongated soft palates which were causing the obstruction.

After the operation, all patients complained of severe throat pain which required strong painkillers. One patient haemorrhaged and had to undergo another operation for this. Nine patients regurgitated food and liquids for around two months, after which time the problem cleared up and did not recur. Five patients had extremely nasal speech after the operation, but again, this was not permanent. No patients developed permanent voice changes.

Now for the most important aspect: what effect did the operation have on their snoring? According to assessment by bedpartners, the snoring levels went down to one – in other words, no snoring at all. When questioned afterwards, all of the patients said that given the choice again they would have definitely had the surgery.

Further results of the follow-up study, obtained by postal questionnaire, were that 91 per cent of the patients experienced either complete relief or dramatic reduction in snoring levels. Mr Gleeson concluded that UPPP is far more satisfactory for heavy snorers than for sufferers from sleep apnoea, but added that all patients should attempt to lose weight before considering embarking on throat surgery. In some cases, weight loss may mean that surgery is no longer needed.

The study of the 22 patients concluded that UPPP was a safe and effective operation and that there were no permanent post-operative complications. It is interesting to reflect that, although male snorers outnumber female snorers by about four to one, UPPP was originally developed to cure a woman's snoring.

Nasal Surgery

In some cases, the snoring may be caused by nasal complications. The commonest of these are polyps in the nasal passages which block the airways. Nasal polypectomy is a simple operation to get rid of these polyps, but again, it should be carried out only after detailed assessment at a sleep laboratory and after X-rays have established that nasal polyps are a significant cause of the snoring.

Nasal polyps are swellings that develop in the lining of the nose and sinuses, usually because of allergy or infection. Although the operation is extremely successful, nasal polyps tend to come back if their root cause is not addressed. Some doctors believe that sufferers from nasal polyps should try to locate the cause of the allergy and treat this before embarking on surgery.

Tracking down allergies can be a complicated and time-consuming business and, ideally, needs specialist assessment at a reputable allergy clinic. At one time, there were very few hospital allergy clinics, and this lack paved the way for get-rich-quick schemes led by unqualified people, who set up their own clinics. When allergy experts at Guy's Hospital tested the claims of some of these private allergy clinics, they found that in every case the clinicians failed to diagnose the correct allergy.

Moral: if you suspect your snoring is being caused by an allergy, or X-rays have established the presence of nasal polyps, ask your doctor for referral to a hospital allergy clinic. There are, at the time of writing, not many in the UK, but their number is growing all the time.

It has been found that wheat and milk allergies are extremely common, and if you suffer from a degree of nasal congestion, simply cutting out these foods from your diet (I say 'simply', but of course it's not so simple as they exist in so many modern foods) may clear up the problem and cure your snoring without any need for nasal surgery.

It's always worth trying non-invasive remedies first, as all surgery constitutes a shock to the system.

Tracheostomy

This is the most severe anti-snoring operation and is rapidly falling into disfavour as UPPP and CPAP units take its place. Before either of these procedures became established, however, tracheostomy was the only treatment available for obstructive sleep apnoea. Nowadays, it is rarely done unless it seems there is absolutely no other option. It is not usually carried out just to stop snoring, but where patients with OSA have life-threatening cardiac problems directly related to their night-time breathing difficulties.

The operation is quite major and consists of opening up the trachea (windpipe) to bypass the upper airways altogether. As the tracheostomy bypasses the natural airway, patients have to learn to live with a tube permanently in their throats. It is like any other 'ostomy' in that there is an opening made in the body, and this in itself can cause complications. Patients have to cover up the tube to speak, and they will never be able to swim again.

People may be referred for tracheostomy if they have already had UPPP and it hasn't worked, as they will not be able to use the CPAP unit after the UPPP operation. Although there are post-operative complications with this operation, most doctors agree that it works well to overcome breathing problems and can be extremely successful in this regard.

It is just as successful as CPAP, but is a far more major procedure and not to be carried out unless there is absolutely no other option.

Other Surgical Procedures

The two other operations which can be used to stop snoring are tonsillectomy and adenoidectomy. But as these operations are more suitable for children, and are rarely carried out with adults, they will be discussed more fully in the Chapter 5.

CHAPTER FIVE

Snoring and Children

Although snoring is usually associated with elderly, overweight men who drink and eat too much, the fact is that children can suffer from snoring as well.

Parents should never ignore their child's snoring, but take it as a sign that something is wrong with the child's breathing. Snoring is not, as some people imagine, part of what the child is like – it is an abnormality and should be attended to without delay.

Unlike adult snorers, or the fat boy in *The Pickwick Papers*, most children who snore are not overweight. By contrast, they are likely to be thin and underweight for their age. They are also likely to have very poor appetites and be slow and picky eaters.

Children should not snore, and it is not normal for them to snore, except perhaps temporarily if they have a cold. So parents should never ignore a child's snoring or expect that the child will eventually grow out of it. Any persistent snoring in children needs medical attention straight away, as childhood snoring can progress to sleep apnoea.

The signs of possible sleep apnoea in children are: loud snoring followed by periods of silence and loud, choking sounds as the child attempts to get his or her breath. The child will be a restless sleeper, difficult to wake up in the morning, and may even wet the bed. This happens because of a reduction in muscle tone when the child is deeply asleep.

Down's Syndrome children are particularly likely to snore, because the anatomical design of their tongues means that their airways are always partially obstructed.

Other children who snore may find it hard to concentrate at school and may even be considered of below average intelligence because they always seem sleepy in the daytime. They are usually underweight and small for their age, and may have small or recessed chins.

These children may breathe with their mouths during the day and have their mouths constantly open, making them look vacant and stupid.

Sometimes, chronic nasal congestion in children may be caused by allergy or infection. If a child snores persistently, this may well be caused by allergic reaction to foods or to the condition of the bedroom. The air in the bedroom should be humid, as having dry nasal membranes can lead to snoring.

It is also worth removing possible sources of allergy in the bedroom, such as feather pillows, wool blankets and animal hairs.

Asthma in children can also lead to snoring.

Try to make sure your child sleeps on his or her side, perhaps by propping him or her up with special pillows. As we have seen, sleeping on the back can often cause snoring.

All the other stop-snoring advice applies to children: don't let them eat big meals late at night just before going to bed, and try to make sure they get some exercise in the daytime.

OPERATIONS TO CURE SNORING

The overwhelming cause of snoring in children is nasal or upper airway obstruction, caused by over-large adenoids or tonsils.

At one time, almost every child had his or her tonsils and adenoids removed, almost as a matter of course. Nowadays, doctors are far more reluctant to perform these operations; even in the old days, most of them probably weren't necessary anyway. But adenoidectomy and tonsillectomy should certainly be considered for any young child who snores at night.

It is always worth trying home remedies before going ahead with any operation. But if there does not seem to be any chronic allergy, and self-help treatments make no difference to the snoring, then adenoidectomy or tonsillectomy – or both – may be recommended.

Both operations are usually highly successful and the loud snoring stops within days of the operation.

Adenoidectomy

This is a minor operation to remove enlarged spongy tissue from the back of the nose. It is recommended for children who suffer from snoring and mouth-breathing because of enlarged adenoids.

Tonsillectomy

This is a minor procedure for children and should be considered when the child suffers from constant colds, breathes through the mouth and is always restless at night. As with adenoidectomy, it should be considered only when other possible causes of snoring have been investigated and eliminated.

After tonsillectomy, the child will suffer from a sore throat for a few days, after which there will be no more adverse symptoms and the snoring usually stops at once. Tonsillectomy may also be recommended for adults who continue to snore, but the procedure is not quite as straightforward as it is for children. Although the operation for adults is identical to that for children, adults do not recover as quickly and can suffer a painful sore throat for up to two weeks afterwards. Also, adult tonsillectomy is not as successful as a snoring cure – and UPPP may have to be performed at the same time.

Some children may grow out of being 'adenoidal' without any treatment and will stop snoring and mouth-breathing naturally. However, now that we know so much about snoring and its possible dangers, it is worth having any persistent snoring investigated. Snoring is *not* normal in anybody.

HYPNOTHERAPY

Some doctors have suggested that hypnosis might be useful for treating children who snore. It seems unlikely, however, that hypnotherapy could treat snoring successfully, as this is above all a physical and not a psychosomatic complaint.

The thing to do with children is to get the snoring investigated first, to determine whether any physical obstruction is causing the problem. It may well be that all the behavioural symptoms which could be seen as psychosomatic, such as bedwetting, poor concentration, lack of appetite and inability to eat properly, are actually caused by the snoring resulting in disturbed sleep night after night.

If the apparent behavioural problems persist after thorough investigation and surgical procedures, then perhaps hypnotherapy could be tried, especially if the child continues to suffer from bedwetting. But always assume that it's the snoring causing the problems, rather than behavioural difficulties. Children do not snore to be awkward, or to get attention.

It is extremely difficult for a child to be bright and alert, to grow properly and to do well at school, if his or her sleep is being disturbed by mouth-breathing and loud snoring night after night. We now know that physical growth and brain repair happen mainly at night during sleep, and that underweight, nervous, tired children are most probably those who are never getting a good night's sleep.

It is also now known that heavy, persistent snoring can cause brain damage – so don't let your child continue to snore. Apart from anything else, a persistently snoring child is likely to be laughed at by other children in the family, be unwelcome to stay in friends' houses and will, in time, suffer from low self-confidence and low self-esteem.

As confidence and self-esteem is always fragile in children anyway, and children are very sensitive to any suggestion that they snore, don't ever let the problem continue without doing anything about it.

CHAPTER SIX

Some Snorers' Stories

Although around 50 per cent of the population snore, at least to some extent, most people consider trying to do something about it only when it has become so bad that it is seriously disrupting social life and relationships – or when a partner or close relative complains about not being able to sleep.

The stories here are of people who fall into this category – and illustrate just how seriously life and health can be disrupted by snoring.

They also show just how effective modern treatments can be, for people who have decided to take their snoring in hand.

Bryan
Bryan, a journalist, has spent most of his professional life as a foreign correspondent on national newspapers. As such, although often working very hard and in dangerous circumstances, he also enjoyed the heavy-drinking, constant partying life of the ex-patriate.

Bryan, now retired from his job on a national Sunday newspaper, tells how asthma, snoring and eventually, severe sleep apnoea led to serious disruption in the quality of his life.

I don't know how many years I had the snoring problem. As a child and young man, I suffered from asthma, and this was why I went abroad to work in the first place, to see whether better and sunnier climates might suit me more.

When I was in my twenties, my lung collapsed. At the time I was newly married and working at the Daily Telegraph *in London. The asthma was very difficult to control and I couldn't breathe very well. I had a weak chest, and seemed to have inherited the asthma from my family. My father had the same complaint.*

Anyway, I thought that a hotter country would help the asthma, and I went with my wife to work in East Africa. The climate there did me a hell of a lot of good, as it was hot and dry. The only problem was that I became allergic to jacaranda trees! But apart from that, there were no problems with my health.

I stayed 12 years there, working as a foreign correspondent, then wondered what to do next. Harold Evans, then editor of the Sunday Times, *asked us to go to Jerusalem, where it was also hot and dry. We went – and I found that the only climatic problem there was the wind.*

Most of the time, I was okay. My health was fine, and we both very much enjoyed the life out there.

Then a tragedy occurred. Bryan's wife died of cancer, leaving him with four young children to bring up, the youngest of whom were twins of six.

For a time, my 17-year-old daughter helped me, but then she went to Philadelphia and got married, so I was left on my own.

I carried on as best I could as a single father for several years, getting up at six in the morning, getting breakfast for the kids, going to the office, picking the kids up from school, cooking their evening meal.

This wasn't too bad if I wasn't too busy, but whenever there were riots to cover, and I had to be away, it was difficult to arrange proper care.

The effect of all this, says Bryan, was that his health got worse and worse.

Of course at the time, I attributed my health problems to stress and having to do too much, but I was by this time very overweight and had high blood-pressure.

Bryan says that he probably snored extremely loudly during this time, but because he was single and sleeping alone, he had no idea how bad the problem had got.

If I had been sleeping with somebody, I expect the snoring problem would have come to light much sooner; but as it was, I didn't know about it and neither did anybody else. I could have been snoring heavily for 15 years and all that time my health was getting steadily worse.

After a time, a woman came to work for Bryan, helping him with the cooking, children and housework.

When I was due to leave Jerusalem to go to South Africa for my next job, she asked to come with me. A relationship developed, which culminated in our marriage.

My wife is American and soon after we got married, she was horrified by my loud snoring. She said, 'Do you mind if I tape it?' – and we found that it was very loud

97

indeed. Being American, she had heard of sleep laboratories, and she knew how serious snoring could be, so she encouraged me to do something about it.

As it was, I didn't do anything about it until the assignment in South Africa came to an end, and we settled back in England. Then my wife said I ought to go to a sleep clinic. Of course, I had never heard of them, and had no idea what to expect.

On his wife's advice, Bryan visited a sleep laboratory on the Grays Inn Road, and loud snoring accompanied by sleep apnoea was confirmed.

Of course, I'd never heard of sleep apnoea and had no idea what it was, although I gathered it was serious. The doctor in charge said that really they ought to operate on the uvula, but in view of my age – 63 – he thought this might be unwise. Also, my long history of asthma decided him against it.

So instead, I was advised to make some lifestyle changes. The first thing, the doctor said, was to get my weight down, and I was given a diet. I've found this extremely difficult to follow, but have managed to lose over a stone.

The other thing, of course, was to cut down the drinking. During my years as a foreign correspondent, I had got used to drinking every evening – everything was an excuse for a party. But now, I only ever drink low-alcohol beers. The doctor told me that if I carried on drinking at the same level, I might die in my sleep. It was also possible that if I hadn't remarried somebody who actually knew something about snoring and sleep apnoea, I might well have died in my sleep anyway, as the apnoea was quite serious.

Bryan says that his main problem all his life has been with mouth-breathing, due to his nostrils often being blocked.

> As surgery was out for somebody of my age, I tried the Nozovent. This has helped and, although I found it irritated at first, I have now got used to it. The only danger comes if I roll over in my sleep, but now I find it quite comfortable.
>
> I haven't tried a CPAP unit yet, as we are seeing whether these other remedies work, but if I have any more problems I will certainly consider using one. I still wake up a lot at night, and tend to sleep well for about four hours before sleeping fitfully. Now that I've retired it's easier because I try to have a nap in the afternoon.

Bryan, now 65, says that he does still snore, but nothing like as loudly as he used to. The sleep apnoea, he said, made him very tired and lethargic during the daytime.

> My wife says that I don't snore when I sleep on my side, but I got into the habit of sleeping on my back.
>
> I was very sharp at one time, and it was after my first wife died that I started to fall asleep in the daytime. I thought that it was my life as a foreign correspondent, plus the strain of looking after the kids, which was responsible for my doziness.
>
> At the time I was drinking a lot of red wine, sherry, brandy, every night, and I couldn't take it. I would often fall asleep during mealtimes. I never actually fell asleep while driving, but I did feel dozy, and when I married again I decided not to drive as I thought I would be unsafe. Now my wife drives me everywhere.

There is no doubt, Bryan says, that snoring and sleep apnoea problems have blighted his professional life.

I just wish now I'd known about the problem 20 years ago, so that I could have done something about it before it got so bad.

Snoring is certainly no joke, as I've learned to my cost. I would now say to anybody who snores: take it seriously, get it investigated, as it really can damage your health. In my case, a lot of damage had been done before I sought any kind of treatment, damage which could probably have been prevented if I'd known about the warning signs years ago.

But in those days, nobody was taking snoring seriously.

Allen Davey

Allen Davey, a chartered builder still in his thirties, is such a loud snorer that he has to sleep at the opposite end of his house from his wife.

Snoring has adversely affected my personal and family life for very many years. I don't smoke but have always had nasal stuffiness and we've even had to move house because of my snoring.

It all started, he says, when he caught whooping cough from his younger daughter.

It took six months for me to get over it, and I couldn't seem to breathe properly at all. Eight years ago, I decided to try and do something about my snoring problem, and I had nasal surgery to try to correct the obstruction. I also tried hypnotherapy, and it did no good at all. The nasal septoplasty, to correct a deviated nasal septum, was also completely unsuccessful.

The only way to stop snoring is in some way to change your anatomy so as to make breathing easier and prevent or overcome the obstruction.

In my case, the solution has been to have a CPAP unit. This is for me the only thing that has been effective at all, and it gives amazingly good sleep. Although its been called the world's most effective contraception, is a nuisance to set up and makes a noise, it's definitely the lesser of two evils.

It gives marvellous results, and you feel a completely different person.

Even so, Allen's snoring has seriously disrupted his marital life. 'I haven't slept in the same room as my wife for years – it would be impossible,' he says.

Allen's own struggles with snoring led him to set up the British Snoring and Sleep Apnoea Association, which runs a helpline for sufferers and also offers a 90-day stop-snoring plan.

A lot of calls come to our helpline because partners won't sleep in the same room as snorers. In many cases, people haven't got spare rooms, so the snorer or the partner has to sleep on the sofa, or come to other makeshift arrangements.

There's no doubt that persistent snoring makes people feel extremely rejected and as if nobody likes them. And that's apart from the difficulties that disturbed sleep and daytime doziness can cause. And it's not always easy to do something about the problem. In a way, the alcohol snorer has it easier, because at least he can choose not to drink. But by no means is all snoring connected with alcohol. Many problems are to do with anatomical design, some kind of obstruction in the nose or throat, or the legacy of an illness, as in my case.

I founded the Association when I looked around for something to help me and found there was nothing. Now, we're doing our best to get the message across that snoring should be taken seriously and that much more research into the subject is needed.

Most of Allen's members are men, although a surprising number are women.

If men are embarrassed by snoring, then women are even more so. To them it seems so unladylike.

Here are two further stories, from women this time, proving that you don't have to be male, elderly or a heavy drinker to have a severe snoring problem.

Pauline

Pauline is a 35-year-old housewife who has suffered from serious, chronic snoring for five years.

My husband complained about it, and it got so bad that often he had to go downstairs and sleep on the sofa.

He would prod me in the ribs and tell me I was snoring, and I often seemed to be wide awake at this point. Of course, I didn't believe my snoring was as bad as he made out, and I put it down to his being an exceptionally light sleeper.

But then he tape recorded the snoring one night, and I could no longer ignore it. It was truly terrible.

When she next went to her doctor, Pauline mentioned the snoring.

My doctor laughed and said she thought nothing much could be done about it, but she did refer me to an ENT specialist at the Radcliffe Infirmary at Oxford.

Really, I only went to the doctor to satisfy my husband that I didn't snore on purpose and that there was nothing whatever that could be done. But to my surprise, the ENT doctor said that my throat was very narrow and was causing breathing obstruction. He sent me for a scan, and this confirmed what he had thought – that I had a very narrow throat and palate, which was causing a sucking noise as I slept.

The ENT surgeon wanted to operate there and then with a UPPP, but I was very sceptical and undecided. After that, though, I spent a night in Dr Stradling's sleep laboratory where I was wired up to lots of machines – and everything was confirmed.

I thought I wouldn't be able to sleep very well in the lab, but to my surprise I did. After my ENT surgeon saw the results of the sleep lab tests, he said he'd like to operate straightaway, so I agreed.

Pauline had the UPPP operation in May 1990 – and hasn't snored since.

From my point of view, the operation has been completely successful. Within a fortnight of having the operation I was completely cured – and my husband hasn't complained once.

I was warned that I might start regurgitating through the nose, but this hasn't been a problem. Occasionally when I laugh food goes up my nose, but very rarely. I can eat socially without any problems, but I have to make sure I don't swallow too quickly.

103

She is now convinced of the great benefits of having snoring properly investigated.

Obviously I didn't think I snored, and was convinced my husband was making out it was worse than it was. But the sleep lab tests confirmed just how loud it was – certainly loud enough to be heard in other rooms.

The benefits have certainly been greater than just stopping my husband from complaining. Without really realizing it, I had very little energy. I was overweight – and since the operation, I have lost a stone and a half without cutting down on food at all, simply because I have so much more energy during the daytime, because I'm sleeping properly at night. I know now that chronic snoring always causes disturbed sleep and that was why I always felt so tired.

Also, for years I had gone to the doctor with my weight problem, saying that I didn't eat much, but couldn't seem to lose any weight. Now, my energy levels are so much higher, and many people have told me I look better and brighter.

Initially, I was very reluctant to have my snoring investigated, and extremely sceptical about the success of any operation to cure the problem. But now I'd recommend anybody who knows he or she snores to go and have it investigated.

Janet

Janet, a 24-year-old trainee accountant, says that her snoring problems were first noticed when she went to live with her boyfriend David.

I don't really know whether or not I snored before that,

but my family never mentioned it. Nor had any friends I went to stay with pointed it out.

But whether it just got worse, or whether everybody had been too polite to say anything, I don't know. But certainly I was never aware of a problem.

But soon after David and I moved in together, he began to complain. At first I thought he was having me on, then he said he would tape record the snores. They were extremely loud, but I was convinced he'd turned the volume up.

Confirmation came when other people living in the same house began to complain as well.

Then I knew that David wasn't making it up. Although I seemed to be deeply asleep, David's sleep was being interrupted. He would wake me up, and as soon as I went back to sleep, I would start snoring again, he said. In the end, he took to sleeping in the spare room, just to get some sleep.

Part of the problem was that I slept on my back. I kept trying to sleep on my side, but I always rolled onto my back. I did all the usual things, like sewing a cotton reel into my nightie, but it had no effect at all.

Eventually, Janet mentioned the problem to her doctor.

By this time, it had become very serious. But I had no idea that anything could be done. To my surprise, my doctor took it all seriously and referred me to a sleep laboratory. He'd obviously had cases like this before.

I spent a couple of nights in the sleep laboratory wired up to all the machines and, of course, hardly snored at all. I think the reason was that the hospital bed was very narrow and I had no difficulty sleeping on my side.

105

Tests and investigations showed that Janet had a narrowed palate, and she was referred for UPPP.

I had the operation to widen the palate, and it certainly helped, but it didn't seem to get to the root of the problem.

The doctor in charge of the sleep laboratory thought I might have enlarged adenoids, but then decided it couldn't be the case at my age. But when he did X-rays, he found that this was in fact the main problem, and I had another operation to remove the adenoids.

Since that time, I haven't snored at all. After the operations, I went to spend another night in the sleep laboratory, and all the machines showed that I was perfectly normal. The operations have made the most incredible difference – and now David never complains at all.

I also find that I am more alive than I used to be. Without really realizing it, I used to go round in a daze. Obviously, I didn't attribute it to disturbed sleep, as I always seemed to sleep so very deeply. It's only after the treatment that I have been aware of the difference.

Before I had the operations, I had no idea that anything could be done about snoring – but now I would advise anybody to go to the doctor, as modern treatments really can be effective, and these days snoring is taken seriously.

CHAPTER SEVEN

Stop-Snoring Inventions

Because snoring drives so many hearers mad, and because there is not, and probably never will be, a simple anti-snoring cure or pill, many scientists and inventors have unleashed their imagination on trying to find a definitive way of stopping the dreadful noise.

Anybody who pays a visit to the Patent Office in London and looks up the snoring prevention devices will find hundreds and hundreds of these, in all languages, from all over the world. The inventions are usually illustrated with highly complicated diagrams that often seem to indicate that the inventor was having such fun creating the design that he or she had forgotten all about the poor human being who might have to use it. Many of the patent devices look exactly like those one might expect to find in a boys' comic – and in many cases, they are about as practical.

Although some Victorians exercised their inventiveness on snoring cures and treatments, interest has certainly hotted up over the past 20 years and every year sees literally dozens and dozens of ingenious devices being granted patents.

The reason 'mad scientists' keep trying to find the definitive cure is obvious: anybody who really could produce a contraption that guaranteed to stop snoring forever would undoubtedly make a vast fortune. In this respect, the search for the anti-snoring cure that really works is rather like the age-old quest for an effective hair restorer – anybody who could absolutely guarantee that the product worked on everybody would very soon be rich.

Unfortunately, what many inventors haven't realized is that snoring has very many causes and that it is unlikely that there ever will be a simple cure, even when everything is known about the reasons for snoring. And most sleep experts say that far more research is needed before anybody will come up with all the answers about snoring.

For very many years, it has been understood that some people's snoring has something to do with mouth-breathing, and that if only a way could be found of keeping the mouth closed during sleep then the snoring would automatically stop. Most of the inventions, it must be said, have concentrated on simply stopping the noise rather than trying to get at the root cause of the snoring.

For instance, it was probably not realized until very recently that overweight and alcohol were two of the main contributors to snoring, or that sometimes, people might have anatomical problems that simply made it impossible for them to breathe properly through their noses.

One American device patented in 1900 consisted of a shoulder brace for keeping the sleeper rigidly on his side. A fierce-looking pronged metal object dug him in the back if ever he tried to sleep in this position, causing extreme pain. Inventions patented in the 1920s by

No. 663,825.

L. E. WILSON.
SHOULDER BRACE AND ANTISNORING ATTACHMENT.

(Application filed Mar. 12, 1900.)

Patented Dec. 11, 1900.

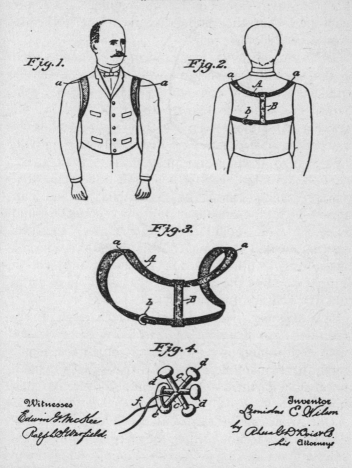

Witnesses
Edwin G. McKee
Ralph G. Warfield.

Inventor
Leonidas C. Wilson
by Chas. B. Dair Co.
his Attorneys

The shoulder brace and anti-snoring attachment patented in 1900.

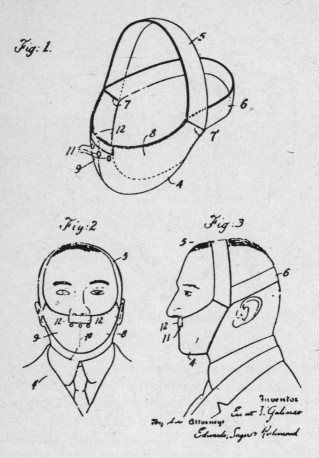

E. V. GALIARDO.
APPARATUS FOR CONTROLLING RESPIRATION.
APPLICATION FILED APR. 4, 1918

1,296,946.

Patented Mar. 11, 1919.

The Galliardo "apparatus for controlling respiration",
patented in 1919.

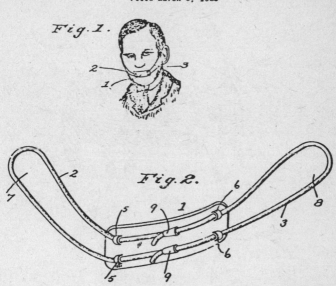

Sept. 16, 1930.

R. GARVEY

1,775,718

MOUTH CLOSING DEVICE

Filed March 5, 1928

The Garvey 'mouth closing device', patented in 1928.

Ernest Galliardo and Richard Garvey are torturous-looking creations for keeping the mouth closed during sleep, thus preventing snoring noises from escaping.

From Victorian times until the 1980s, most anti-snoring implements concentrated on keeping the mouth closed at night. One patented in October 1979 by Charles F. Samuelson is a gruesome-looking contraption that the snorer wears in his mouth. The

111

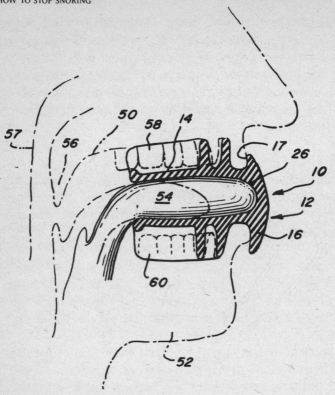

The Samuelson 'anti-snoring and anti-bruxism device', patented in 1979.

device clamps firmly over the teeth – to put the tongue in a forward position and prevent it from occluding the oropharynx.

The inventor describes his device thus:

> *The device . . . is an integrally molded body providing an*
> *externally located lip-engaging member and internally*

located parts to be positioned within the user's mouth. The internal portion of the device provides dental engaging arches and a rearwardly-opening central socket for co-operating with the forward portion of the user's tongue in a manner to draw the tongue forwardly so as to increase the unobstructed dimension of the nasal breathing passage.

The invention, Mr Samuelson goes on to say, 'substantially eliminates oral breathing,' and facilitates nasal breathing. An additional feature of this device, according to its inventor, is that it eliminates nocturnal tooth-grinding as well.

In 1971, another American, Sigmund H. Ancerewicz, Jr, patented an invention for collecting drainage from the tracheal openings for people who had undergone tracheostomies – the standard operation for terrible snoring before UPPP was perfected. Again, the device looks gruesome in the extreme.

Very many anti-snoring gadgets come from Australia. Whether snoring is very much worse there, or whether Australians are just more inventive, is not known – but certainly they have exercised all their ingenuity in this area.

As we have seen, until the 1970s, most anti-snoring devices consisted of contraptions to keep the mouth closed during the night. But with the dawning of the electronic age, even more ingenious machines have been invented to stop snoring.

By the time the electronic devices came into being, inventors had also assimilated a modicum of psychology and took into account such things as

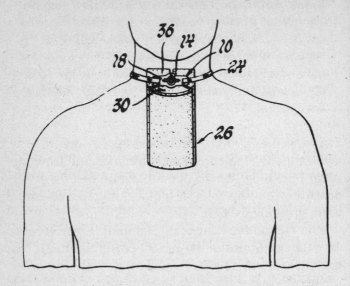

The Ancerewicz 'tracheostomy device', patented in 1971.

behavioural conditioning when perfecting their inventions.

An Australian anti-snoring device patented in 1984 was a small battery-powered miniaturized machine that fitted into the ear of the sleeper to wake him up when he started snoring. The object of the invention was to 'provide a compact anti-snoring device which can be worn comfortably in the ear of the sleeper and which provides an aversive but not dangerous stimulus.' There were no wires or straps in this device, so it could be used when travelling, camping, and so on.

It was, apparently, comfortable to wear, and the

electrical shock that resulted when snoring noises were picked up were not dangerous in any way. In addition, the device did not disturb the snorer's bedpartner. The inventor realized that after a time snorers might become habituated to the noise the machine made and would ignore it when asleep. So the device was made to be self-adjusting so that ever-louder noises could be emitted.

The device looked rather like a hearing aid and was supposed to work on the Pavlovian principle that the snorer could eventually learn to stop the noise which caused the buzz in his ear, i.e. to stop snoring. There does not seem to have been any allowance made for the fact that most snorers are completely unaware of their snoring – and cannot stop it by a simple act of will.

An early American electronic anti-snoring device consisted of a neck band worn by the sleeper which comprised an electrical circuit that detected the snore and then imparted a high-voltage shock to condition the sleeper against snoring in future.

Another American invention woke up the sleeper by shaking the pillow when he started to snore. The Australians also introduced a device consisting of a box located under the mattress which induced the pillow to move, thus allowing the snorer to change position without waking up.

There was also about this time, the early eighties, a tape recorder invented in the US which was actuated by the sound of snoring to play back a pre-recorded message to the sleeper via an earplug.

The earplug was connected to the tape recorder by a cord, and it was all very complicated. There was also

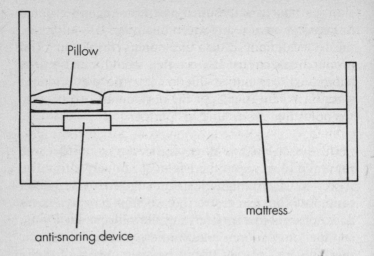

Pillow

mattress

anti-snoring device

A box under the mattress would move the snorer's pillow in response to his snoring, thereby making him change sleeping position.

the possible danger that the sleeper could become entangled in the cord, or that the earplug could become dislodged if the sleeper tossed and turned during the night.

Another conditioning device patented around this time consisted of a visual display unit which registered and reported the number of times the sleeper snored loudly during the night.

A Swedish device consisted of two electrodes worn as a bracelet around the wrist which gave a small electric shock when the sleeper snored. The idea of this device was that the electric shocks induced the sleeper to change his sleeping position to one in which he did not snore.

In the 1970s and 1980s, according to patents granted or pending, very many inventors in the US, Australia, the UK, Germany, China and Japan concentrated on producing electronic devices that would wake up the snorer, activate him to the fact that he was snoring, then allow him to change his position and go back to sleep without disturbing his partner.

The success of these inventions has, for the most part, been extremely short-lived, as they are so complicated to wear and in addition are seen as not very attractive. Also, like the mouth-closing devices of the earlier generation of inventors, the electronic contraptions never addressed the root cause of snoring. Now that snoring is so much better understood, and we know that lifestyle changes can very often prevent snoring altogether, there is less need to resort to these 'cures'.

In any case, before considering using a device which closes the mouth, you should be sure that you can breathe unobstructedly through the nose. People usually breathe through the mouth when there is some nasal obstruction, so it is worth getting this seen to before considering devices that keep the mouth shut mechanically.

If you are persuaded to try an electronic device, remember that being wired up can restrict your movements while asleep and mean that you get into abnormal or constricted positions. The CPAP unit, which does of course wire people up to a machine, has been developed as a life-saving device – and is intended only for people who have had sleep apnoea diagnosed.

Otherwise, it is far better to try to ascertain the root

cause of the snoring. The point about all devices is that they only stop snoring when they are being used – they don't actually cure the condition.

If you know you are a chronic snorer, try to find out what is causing you to have disturbed sleep in this way. Many of the mouth-closing and electronic devices actually make sleep more disturbed by waking you up throughout the night, or making you so uncomfortable that you can't sleep properly anyway.

The whole point of stopping snoring is to get a good night's sleep – so don't fall for any exaggerated claims that this or that patent cure can stop snoring forever.

Conclusion

Thanks to intensive research by sleep experts over the past few years, we now know much about snoring, what causes it and what can be done to stop it. In view of this, the days when snoring was considered an embarrassing complaint that nobody would own up to are, with any luck, almost over.

Although snoring has been a favourite subject for cartoonists over the years, and snorers are usually depicted as overweight, unattractive slobs, the fact is that snoring can affect anyone.

Although snoring in older people will almost always be connected to eating and particularly to drinking habits, it is also frequently caused by anatomical defects or deformities which may not come to light until they are properly investigated. Young people who snore and who are not overweight will very probably have some anatomical problem which can be cleared up with a simple operation.

I hope that this book will give hope to all those who snore, or who are told that they snore and are convinced that nothing can be done about the noise, or that their partners or neighbours are wildly exaggerating.

Even if investigations indicate that partners *have* been

exaggerating the noise levels, at least you will know this – and have objective evidence about your snoring. Nobody who is told, or who has reason to believe, that he or she is a chronic snorer, should ever ignore this, or imagine that the problem will clear up by itself.

The chances are that it will get worse unless treated – but these days you can be sure that sympathetic treatment is available.

If your doctor is one of the old school who just laughs at snoring, then show him or her this book – and ask to be referred to an ENT specialist or sleep laboratory.

In the UK, there are now very many sleep laboratories attached to large general hospitals, and their number is growing all the time as it comes to be realized just how important to health, energy levels and daytime functioning a good night's sleep is. Sleep experts will not always recommend operations or being wired up to machines – they would far rather see whether some lifestyle changes will be enough to result in silent nights.

We know now that most people need seven-and-a-half to eight hours' good sleep in order to fulfil their intellectual potential, to remain healthy and to keep their immune system strong.

Although some people, such as former British Prime Minister Margaret Thatcher, may boast that they can function on four or five hours' sleep, the fact is that for the majority of us, this amount is simply not enough to enable us to remain alert all day.

It makes sense to take whatever steps are necessary to ensure that you – and your partner – get optimum rest and refreshment from the time you spend in bed asleep.

As we have seen, snoring can seriously disrupt intimate relationships. It can be difficult to continue to love somebody who keeps you awake night after night with his or her snoring, or whose snoring levels are so high that the only solution seems to be to isolate either the snorer or yourself.

Snoring seriously disrupts the sleep of both the snorer and the bedpartner – which means that both of you are constantly being short-changed on this vital restorative function.

Although there is not one simple stop-snoring nostrum available, there are now enough treatments and cures, both self-help and medical, to ensure that snoring does not continue to be a problem.

If you are a snorer, you owe it to yourself to get a good night's sleep. If you are the partner of a snorer, you also deserve to sleep properly – so don't let the noise continue. Bedpartners *owe* it to the snorer to mention the snoring and offer to work together to try to overcome the problem. Simply digging partners in the ribs, shouting at them, or complaining in the morning does no good at all, as they can't help the snoring, or overcome it by good intentions.

To sum up, snoring is not a character defect, a personality or behavioural problem, but a noise caused by a physical obstruction in the nose or throat. Regard it in the same way you would regard any other health problem – as something to be healed and prevented. It is *not* inevitable as we get older, and it is *not* normal.

We are not designed to snore, but to breathe easily and naturally through the nose, and to sleep peacefully and silently.

121

Glossary of Essential Terms

Adenoidectomy: Surgical removal of the adenoids

Adenoids: Spongy tissues situated in the area behind the nose

Apnoea: Cessation of breathing at night lasting for 10 seconds or more

Collapsible airway: The soft tissues in the upper respiratory tract, which have no rigid support

CPAP unit: Continuous Positive Airway Pressure unit – a high-tech device by which constant air pressure is delivered at night through a mask.

Deviated septum: Injury or anatomical defect causing the cartilage between the nostrils to become twisted, thus causing breathing obstruction

Narcolepsy: Excessive sleepiness during the daytime, caused by problems in the central nervous system

Nasal polypectomy: Surgical removal of polyps in the nose

Pharynx: The cavity situated behind the nose, mouth and larynx

Sinuses: The spaces containing air situated near the nasal cavities

Sinusitis: Infection or inflammation of the mucous membrane lining of the sinuses

Uvula: The flap of flesh hanging from the middle of the soft palate

Uvulopalatopharyngoplasty (UPPP): Surgery to enlarge the air passages at the back of the throat

Resources

Further Reading

Snoring and What to Do About It – a handy leaflet produced by the Sleep Disorders Clinic, Leicester General Hospital, LE5 4PW.

Suppliers

Inphormed Ltd (producers of the *Nozovent*)
Worthy Park House
Abbots Way
Winchester
Hants SO21 1AN
Tel: 0962 87811

Medipost (suppliers of the *Snorestop* pillow)
100 Shaw Road
Oldham
Lancs OL1 4AY
Tel: 061-678 0233
Fax: 061-627 4401

Support Groups

UK
The British Snoring and Sleep Apnoea Association
(BSSAA)
'The Steps'
How Lane
Chipstead
Surrey CR5 3LT
Tel: 0737 557997
(Send large sae for details)

The Insomnia and Snoring Cure Group
Puncheston
Dyfed
SA62 5RN
Wales
(Send sae for details)

USA
The American Sleep Disorders Association
604 Second Street SW
Rochester, MN
55092

Canada
Sleep Disorders Clinic
Foothills Hospital
University of Calgary
Calgary, Alberta
T2N 2T9

Australia
Sleep Centre
Department of Medicine
University of Sydney
NSW 2006

New Zealand
Sleep Disorders Clinic
Department of Neurophysiology
Auckland Hospital
Auckland

South Africa
Sleep Disorders Clinic
Department of Internal Medicine
University of Orange Free State
Bloemfontein 9300

Index

127